YOUR SELF-HEALING POWER

Simple Strategies to Help You Fight Cancer and Other Illnesses

ALINA MANLEY

Balboa Press books may be ordered through booksellers or by contacting:

Balboa Press
A Division of Hay House
1663 Liberty Drive
Bloomington, IN 47403
www.balboapress.com
1 (877) 407-4847

ISBN: 978-1-5043-8669-2 (sc)
978-1-5043-8670-8 (e)

Library of Congress Control Number: 2017913016

Print information available on the last page.

Balboa Press rev. date: 09/13/2017

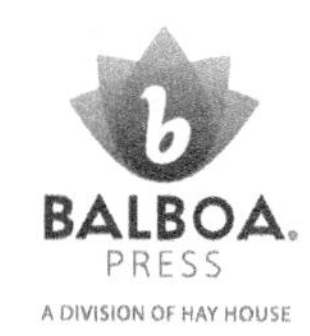

ACKNOWLEDGEMENT

I wish to thank Marianna Kajut who provided the initial translation from the first Polish version of my book. There have been many changes and additions, but Marianna's work was an important base for me.

A very special "Thank you" to my daughter Gosia Bagley, my husband Michael Manley, and my friend Jerry Thompson, who helped edit and compile this work. Their support was crucial.

PREFACE

Wouldn't it be beautiful if we could free ourselves from stress and enhance our ability to heal our body, mind, and spirit in a simple, fast, and effective way? I am going to share with you some practices and techniques that I have learned from my experience as a nurse and a healer, which will help you do just that.

I was inspired to write this book by Stephanie, an oncology patient suffering from leukemia. She was very sick and extremely exhausted after a series of chemotherapies, when a psychologist she knew gave her a book about body-mind work designed to improve one's health. Unfortunately, Stephanie was riddled by fever, nausea, vomiting, and diarrhea and was unable to understand anything she read. The book, however excellent and beautifully written, was too difficult for her to grasp in her condition.

One day she asked me to read her a small chapter of that book. She was so sick that she could not read anything by herself. As I read, she asked for explanations. I saw her determination to fight for life, so I set the book aside and explained to her in simple words how she could boost her ability to heal herself. I taught her basic methods of relaxation, meditation, and visualization. I told her about the energy system in the human body, around the body, and in the Universe. I showed her how to work with her life energy field to restore a better state of health. Our beginning was not easy, as she was very sick and exhausted. I worked with her slowly, step by step, until she got better. Later she continued on her own with minimal help from me. With new levels of strength and hope, Stephanie successfully won the fight for her life.

One day, she asked me, "Why don't you write a book? You should write a short, simple book, which can be understood and used by people like me. You can help many people this way." After a couple of years of writing, editing, and making additions, the book is finally ready. It contains straight-forward descriptions of some very simple and effective techniques to support healing and promote a return to health.

Whether you are suffering from cancer, another serious illness, or simply want to increase your chances of staying healthy throughout your life, the methods included here will greatly help you on your path. You will discover the power of your thoughts and emotions, your ability to use the life energy that surrounds you, and other techniques within your reach that can help you fight illnesses. I hope you enjoy reading and benefit from practicing the described strategies.

Alina Manley

TABLE OF CONTENTS

ACKNOWLEDGEMENT iii

PREFACE v

INTRODUCTION ix

THE POWER OF THOUGHTS 1

THE POWER OF EMOTIONS 7

RELAXATION 13

VISUALIZATION 23

ENERGY POWER OF YOUR BODY 33

TAPPING OR EFT: EMOTIONAL FREEDOM TECHNIQUE 65

OTHER USEFUL STRATEGIES 77

BIBLIOGRAPHY 85

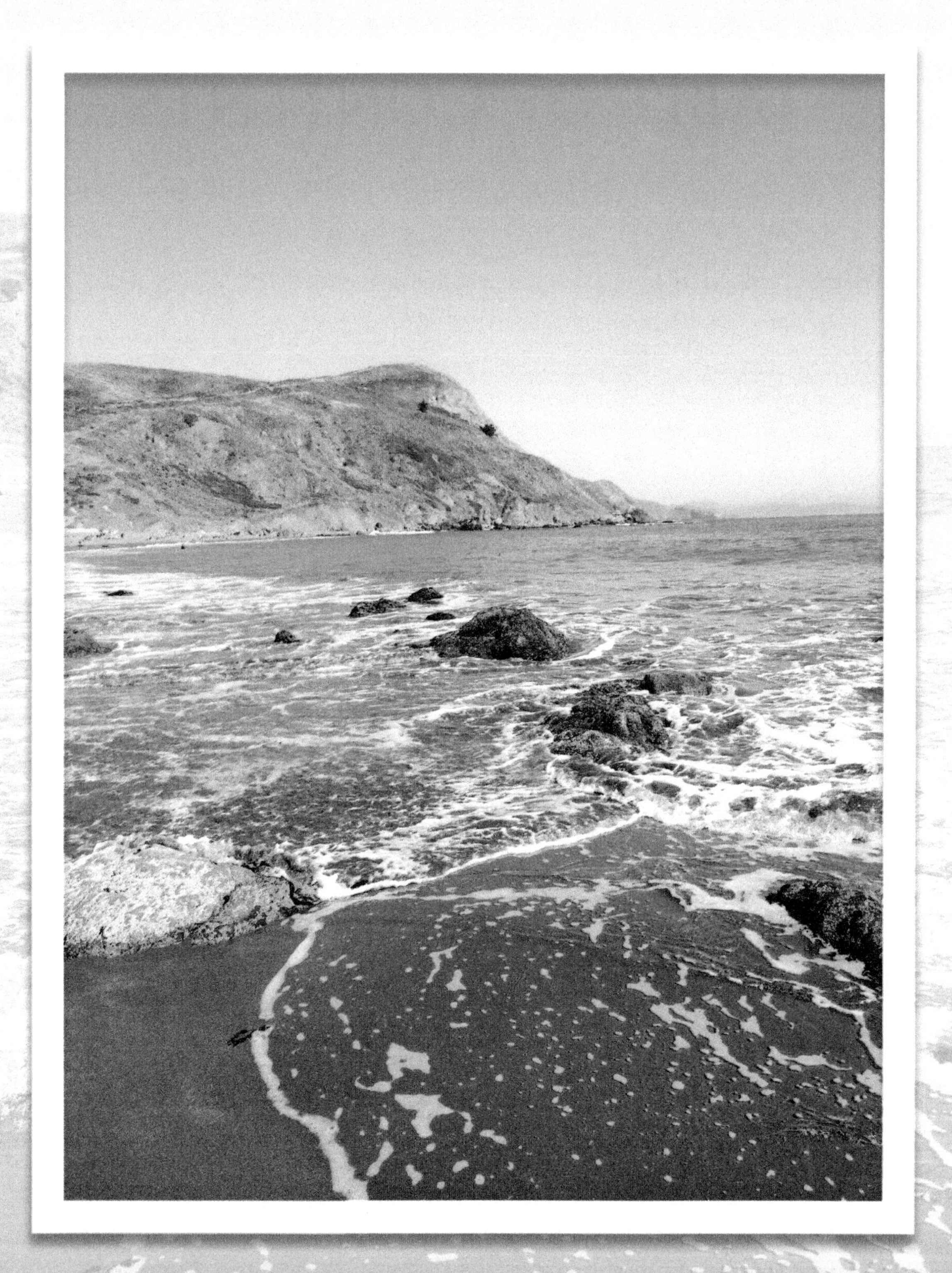

INTRODUCTION

The methods described in this book are neither new nor groundbreaking. Most of them have been used for thousands of years, as the art of healing is as old as human history. Sensitive, gifted people with great compassion and willingness to help others have inhabited all corners of our planet throughout all times. They carried various names in various lands and cultures: magician, holy man, shaman, kahuna, granny woman, midwife, wise woman, wise man, priest, healer, and so on. Written references of healing have been found in Sumerian records left on clay tablets (in cuneiform writing) dated 2200 BC. Other written sources were found in Babylonian, Assyrian, and Egyptian excavations. In India and many parts of Asia, Buddhism has had a huge impact on healing traditions, encouraging meditation, visualization, and physical exercise to promote proper energy flow in the body. In China about 2000 BC, healers used massage, hydrotherapy, and developed acupuncture. They knew the importance of hygiene, diet, and exercise. Native Americans, including the Aztecs, Incas, and Mayas, were excellent herbalists and used various types of healing rituals. They tried to live in harmony with nature. Healers in Europe used herbs and the practice of laying on of hands. All of these ancient techniques have been enriched and mastered through the centuries of practice, and today we can use all these methods and combine them for the best healing results.

My role has been to choose and simplify certain techniques, so they can be easily and effectively used by anyone and anywhere, even by very sick patients in a hospital setting. It is my pleasure to give you these "power tools" to improve your health. I hope that the techniques that you learn from my book help you, just as they helped Stephanie and many others. The "power" which you will utilize is within you! When you get back on your feet, feel free to explore these methods in greater depth - it is well worth the effort.

In the meantime, let's start your journey to health.

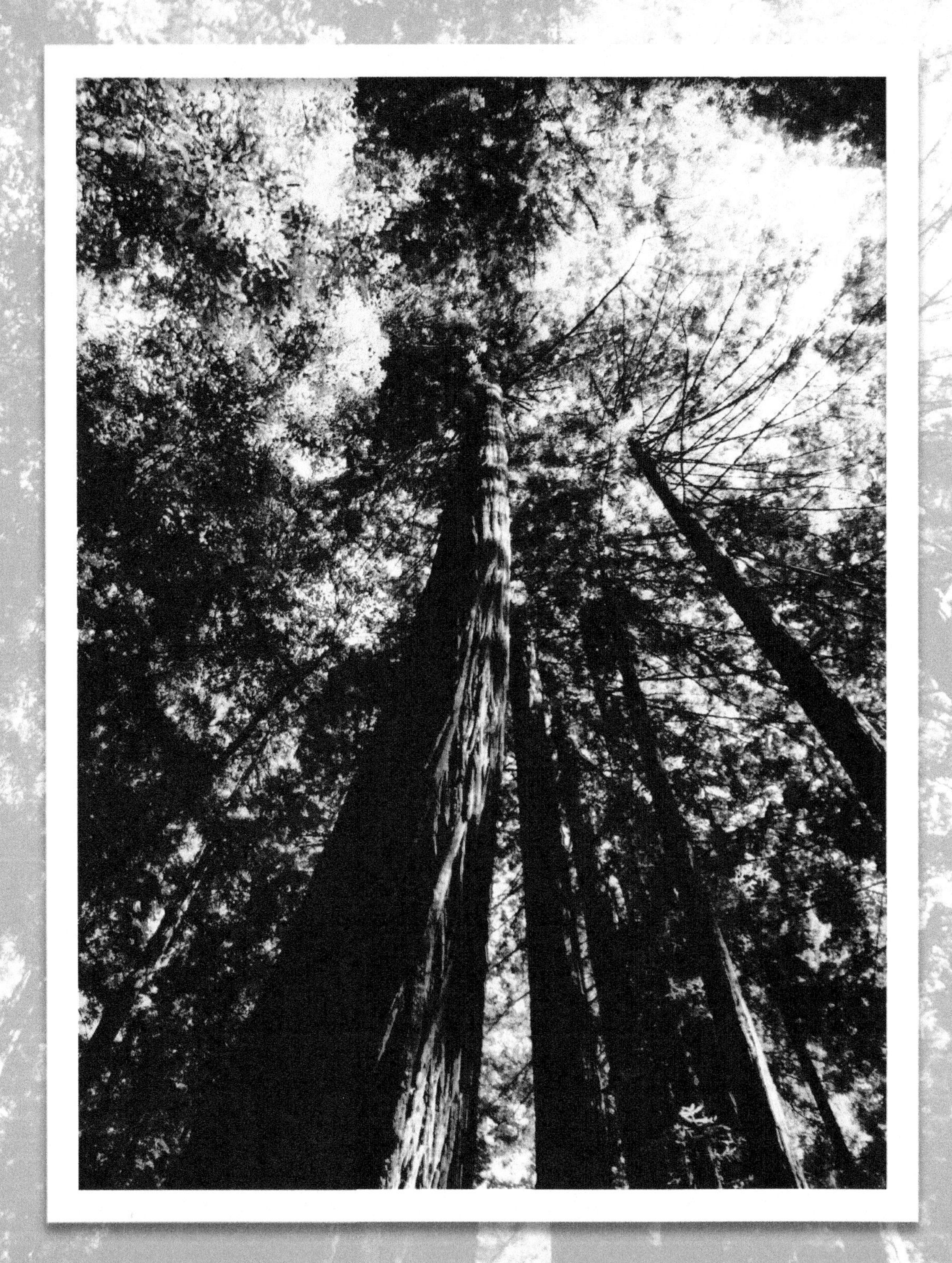

THE POWER OF THOUGHTS

In order to feel better, get back to health, or prolong your lifespan, you need not only good medical care, but you must also be the "Managing Director" of your health. Nobody can make you healthy without your active involvement. You might be surprised when I tell you that your attitude, the way you think about yourself and your health can influence your well-being and quality of life. Do you know that your body can be programmed by your thoughts?

When you wake up in the morning thinking "What horrible weather, the air pressure is low, I am going to have a headache," there is a good chance that your headache is just around the corner. In this case, your body has been programmed by your thoughts to have a headache. However, you can easily change this scenario. Next time, just think, "The weather might not be the best, but I am feeling great, and I'm going to have a good day." Try it. It works.

One day, my friend Anna came for a visit. She had a cold and was feeling a bit under the weather, so she asked me to give her something to alleviate her symptoms. I gave her vitamin C and calcium tablets. I told her what I was giving her, but I suspect she did not pay attention in that moment. That night I was awakened by a phone call from the local

ER. The doctor on duty told me that Anna had an allergic reaction to something, perhaps the medication I gave her. I told the doctor what I gave her. When the doctor explained to Anna that she was given vitamin C and calcium, the allergy symptoms disappeared, and she felt much better. All tests came out negative. After a few hours of observation, she was released from the ER. In this case, Anna's thoughts about an "allergic reaction" were so strong that they caused physical symptoms.

In general, a patient's attitudes play an important role in the results of his or her treatment. I will give you some examples.

"John" had undergone a simple surgery, an uncomplicated appendectomy, and should have been released from the hospital in 1 or 2 days. He was unhappy about everything: an uncomfortable bed, unsatisfactory food, and a bad view from the window. He did not want to get out of bed or turn from one side to the other, even though it was in his best interest. John refused to take his medications. He developed all possible complications, including bedsores, pneumonia, and a blood clot. His stay in the hospital was extended enormously. With a great struggle his medical team brought him back to health.

"Roger" found out he had lung cancer, which spread to his liver and bones. His oncologist gave him very little chance to survive. It was the end stage of the disease with a very poor prognosis. Chemotherapy could prolong his life by only a few months. However, Roger really wanted to see his children reach adulthood and become self-sufficient. He took the small chance that was allotted to him, and turned it into a "power ball" win over his disease. His focus on using all the time he had to prepare his children to become independent was enough to activate the self-regulating, self-healing power of his body; it allowed him to overcome his illness.

"Ted" made a very risky decision in the treatment of his cancer. He refused to undergo surgery and chemotherapy. He chose to use the time he had left to realize his dream – a journey around the world. He sold his house and spent all his savings. He returned after four months, happier than ever. Making his dream come true proved to be the best therapy for him. Tests showed that he was cancer free. He had no house or money, but it did not matter – he was cancer free. He found a new job and began a more conscious and happy new life. He was beaming, and his optimism was contagious.

"Michelle" found out that she had ovarian cancer, just after she discovered that her husband had an affair. She used her illness as a tool to keep her husband. She was happy that her husband felt guilty about his affair, and that he spent all his free time with her, and he was again her kind and loving husband. But this "happiness" did not help in her fight for life.

You might know family members or friends who use their illness as a tool of manipulation to obtain rewards they want. Some people subconsciously feel safe with their unhealthy condition for a number of different reasons. It might be a way for them to get attention, love, a sense of stability, or to gain control over others.

The variations of these kinds of stories are too numerous to recount here. They are a great illustration of the need to start thinking positively and to be honest with yourself. Simply put, your way of thinking has a great influence on your life and health.

To begin looking more closely at your attitudes and thought patterns, start to pay attention to the words you use each day. Try your best to use positive words, even when expressing negative states of being. Instead of the word "bad," try to use the word "well" with a negation right before it. For example, when you don't feel well, try to say "I don't feel well" instead of "I'm feeling awful." The subconscious, which greatly affects your body functions, does not recognize negatives. In the above example, the subconscious will recognize only words like "well" or "awful." Therefore, use only positive terms. Also, try to use the phrase "I choose" rather than "I should." The word "should" often implies guilt, fear, or shame. In place of saying "I should exercise," try to say "I choose to exercise" instead. Another example is saying "I choose to eat better" rather than "I should eat better."

Obviously positive thinking alone is not enough, but it is a very good start, and it is the first step toward better health. Even if you feel you are in a hopeless situation or if you are not in the best health, find something good and beautiful in your life and use it as a bridge to a better future.

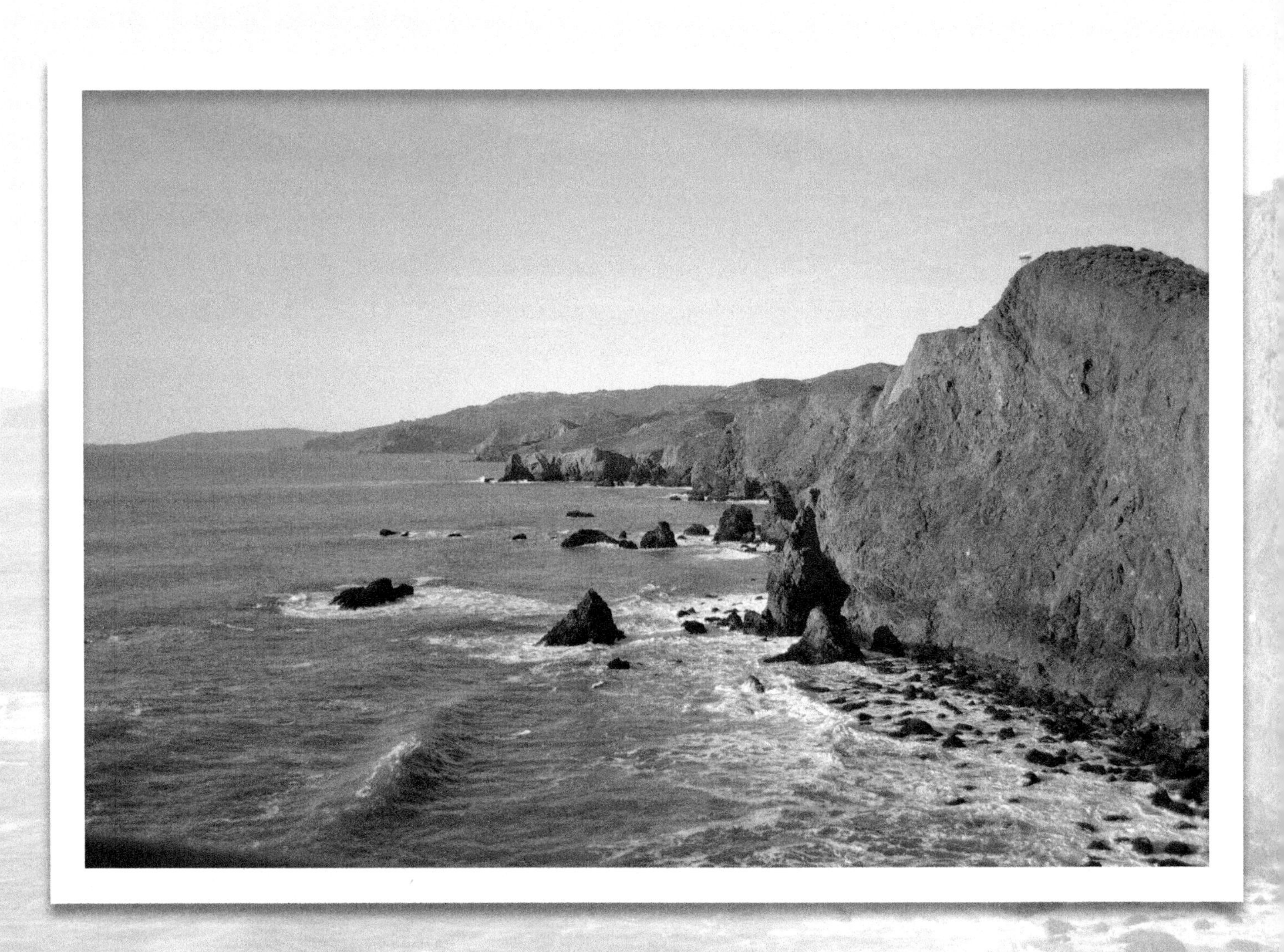

THE POWER OF EMOTIONS

Emotions are another big factor in your life that can influence your health. Negative emotions have the power to lower your immune response, your energy level, and your ability to make wise decisions. On the flip side, if you cultivate positive emotions, you have more of a chance to stay healthier. This is not about pretending to be more positive, but about working through your emotions and resolving the tension. When you are angry, you don't have to deny it or bottle it up. It is best to be aware of the negative or destructive emotion, understand why you feel this way or what caused it, work with it, and find a resolution.

When we receive bad news, when our life, health, career, or safety is endangered and we cannot believe it, we often ask "Why is this happening to me?" This is often the case with patients diagnosed with a serious illness. Sometimes we feel deep resentment, anger, or sadness. Sometimes we blame ourselves, our family, or somebody else. Sometimes we interpret an illness or a misfortune as punishment. It turns out that these emotions are not helpful at all.

There is nothing as destructive as resentment, anger, and self-pity. These negative emotions only worsen your situation. Life has given you an unpleasant surprise. It is unfortunate and largely out of your control.

Instead of dragging yourself down and drowning in despair, it is far more helpful to think about how to get through the situation. Giving up smoldering resentment and suffocating anger is not an easy feat, but you can do it.

Think of the many ways in which you can support yourself through the recovery process instead of pulling yourself down. Think of what you can do to make your treatment more successful. Imagine your sorrow, hate, anger, or self-pity as a huge ball you have to drag behind you. It is heavy, painful, and works like poison. Do you need this kind of extra baggage? I don't think so. It is time to cut the chain that attaches you to this ball of negative emotions. In order to walk freely and easily in this life, you must leave this dark heaviness behind. It is time to move on.

There is a simple exercise I learned that can help you free yourself from your attachment to negative emotions. It involves sending loving energy to someone who hurt you, to someone against whom you hold a grudge, or to someone towards whom you feel anger or hatred. Start to think about a pleasant aspect of this person. He or she may have an attractive smile, nice eyes, beautiful clothes, or some charming personal quality. Concentrate on one good aspect of that person, and try to send him or her loving thoughts. This act can free you from destructive emotions.

One not-very-young lady, when asked if she was ready to forgive her abusive father, said "No, never. This anger defined my life. Who will I be without this feeling? My life will be empty." In another case, a man lost all his savings due to a dishonest financial advisor. This man said that the only pleasure he had was thinking about revenge. He created in his mind multiple scenarios in which there were bad endings for this financial advisor. He did not want to forgive, because the constant thinking about a bad ending for the advisor gave him satisfaction.

Taking this approach keeps people attached to old wounds and poisonous emotions that harm them. They keep themselves in the position of a victim. To start the healing process, you have to stop being a victim. Cut the chain and release the ball of negative emotions. Free yourself of the negativity by practicing **forgiveness.** If there is someone you hate, blame, or consider responsible for your problems, forgive him or her. **Forgiveness benefits you much more than your enemy.**

Dr. Wayne Dyer, a well-known author and speaker, related on many occasions how for many years he carried with him negative emotions about his father who had abandoned his family. He searched for his father in order to confront him about his abandonment of his wife and three sons. He wanted to tell his father how much he hated him. Eventually Dr. Dyer found himself at his father's grave, where he told his father, "...From this moment on, I send you only love..." This was a defining moment for Dr. Dyer. This change in his heart, this act of forgiveness changed the trajectory of his entire life and work.

All of us must cope with life's struggles as best we can. No one is without failure, sin, or mistakes. No one is perfect. So, be gentle with others and yourself. Forgive others and yourself. Enrich your life with love, kindness, compassion, good humor, and laughter. Instead of complaining, try to exercise gratitude. No, do not try – just do it! More positive emotions and thoughts will result in more positive changes in your life. Do not be afraid. It will be a new, fascinating experience, a fresh chapter in your life.

Many of us are tormented by thoughts along the lines of "if only I had made a different decision, if I had taken the other road, if only I was eating healthier." Please stop speculating. It is what it is. Think what you can do now to improve your situation. Think clearly about which problem you can address today. Think about it without emotions. Imagine that "your problem" is not yours but someone else's. This will give you a chance to see your problem from a distance and will improve your ability to find the best solution.

In time, you will be able to distance yourself from negative emotions and thoughts. And this will improve your health and your own ability to help your body heal itself.

Now, let's move to the next step on your path to self-healing: relaxation.

RELAXATION

One of the most important and easiest self-healing techniques is relaxation. It helps individuals regain mental stability, releases the negative effects of stress, and can speed up one's return to health. It can be a starting point for meditation, visualization, and various self-healing techniques or it can work effectively by itself. There are significant benefits and no negative side effects.

All methods of relaxation are good. If you already have some experience and know what form of relaxation you like the most, use it. The method I recommend is very simple, available to anyone, anywhere, and anytime. You don't need special preparation. One general rule is that whatever you do, do it naturally, and don't work too hard.

In all relaxation techniques, you can distinguish three main stages:

1. Deep breathing with full exchange of air in the lungs.
2. Progressive muscle loosening.
3. Quieting of the mind.

Here is a step-by-step guide for each of the stages:

Breathing

We all breathe without thinking about breathing. We just breathe automatically and that is how it should be. By focusing on breathing, you can shift your attention and have an opportunity to free yourself from part of your stress. When you are ill, in pain, or under stress, you need more oxygen, which in turn provides your body with more energy. You can supply your body with extra energy by breathing deeper and slower.

Assume a position that you find comfortable. You can lie down, sit, or stand up, as long as your spine is as straight as possible. Once in your spot, focus your attention on breathing. Inhale and exhale through your nose. Inhale slowly, and gradually fill your abdomen, stomach, and chest with air, until you feel a slightly raised pressure in your arms and head. And now, exhale slowly, releasing the air from chest, stomach, and abdomen. Exhale at the same speed at which you inhaled. If you counted to six while breathing in, also count to six while breathing out. In time you will be breathing deeper and slower. Do not rush it. Start slowly, at your own pace. There is usually a short break between each inhale and exhale. It is very personal. It can take 1-4 seconds. Don't force yourself to breathe deeper or slower than you can. Just find your own pace.

Ten deep breaths are usually enough to oxygenate the body well and to exchange all the air in your lungs. Dizziness may indicate an excess of oxygen. If you start feeling light headed, return to regular breathing.

If you find this kind of breathing difficult, there is a way to make it more manageable. Put your hand on your belly. Breathe in and direct all air down to your belly. While your belly fills with air, your hand will be lifted. Then fill up your chest, hold it for a few seconds, feel it, then exhale, starting from the top of your chest down to your belly. Your hand will now be much closer to your back. This collapsing of the belly will force out the air from the lower part of the lungs, enabling a total exchange of the air in your lungs.

Progressive Muscle Loosening

Releasing muscle tension will restore the correct energy flow in your body, which will have a great effect on stress release, on your health, and well-being. When you are under stress, you usually don't realize how tight your muscles are. It is only when you feel pain in your back, head, or shoulders that you notice something is wrong. You don't have to wait for pain to know that you are under stress. If you know how to control your muscle tension, you will be able to eliminate the effects of stress before they emerge.

The process is easy. First, consciously tense a muscle, and then consciously relax it. The key is to notice the difference between a tense and a loosened muscle. Do it with all the muscles, one by one.

- Start with your facial muscles. Wrinkle your forehead until it hurts, and release it. Note the difference between the tense and relaxed forehead.
- Now, close your eyes. Close your eyes tightly for a moment. Feel the pressure, and release. Then focus on the difference between the two feelings.
- Do the same with the muscles around your lips. Work on facial expressions like an actor. Be very aware of the difference between the feeling of those muscles being tense and then relaxed.
- Migraines usually start with stiff jaws, so don't forget this area. Clench your teeth, feel the muscles strain, relax them consciously. What a relief!
- Raise your shoulders up, very high, all the way up to your ears. Do you feel them stiffen? Does it hurt? That is good, that is how it should feel. Now release them and feel the difference.
- Try to make your shoulder blades touch each other. Pull your elbows backward, with the shoulder blades as close together as possible. Hold it, then slowly relax, and feel the difference.
- Suck in your belly close to your spine, hold it, release, and note the difference.

- Clench your buttocks, hold, and relax. Can you feel the difference?
- Squeeze your fists till you feel the muscles of your arms and forearms tighten. Hold them. Are they shaking? That is good. Relax, and remember the difference.
- Curl your toes down under your feet tight, so tight that you can feel all the muscles in your thighs and calves strained. Then relax them slowly and notice the difference.

Loosening your muscles brings relief from tension and releases some amount of your stress. Now you are ready for the most important part of relaxation: the quieting of your mind.

Quieting of Your Mind

The human mind is usually very busy with various thoughts and it is often very difficult to quiet it down. You are not able to eliminate all thoughts completely, but to calm and focus your mind, you can direct your attention to one object, place, event, or emotion, and gently move the rest of your thoughts into the background.

Do not fight your thoughts. Do not throw them out of your head purposefully, because they will come back like a boomerang. Do not concentrate on getting rid of unwanted thoughts. This will attract them even more. Try your best to let the unwanted, busy thoughts just flow through your mind like clouds through the sky. Let them go, like the wind. Just notice they are here, and let them go.

The following exercise is an easy way to calm the mind down. After you have finished the breathing exercise and the progressive loosening of the muscles, transport your thoughts to your "happy place." Draw from your memory a place and time associated only with good moments and feelings of safety and love, then concentrate and contemplate on this memory. Try to go deeper than just recalling the memory; make the memory alive. The most popular choices for this exercise are memories associated with vacations near the ocean and memories from childhood. If you can find a moment like this in your memory, relive this happy moment using all your senses. Remember the smell of the air, feel the warmth of the sun on your skin, hear the wind blowing, see the colors of the water and the sky, touch the sand, and immerse yourself in serenity.

If you don't remember any beautiful moments in your life, imagine a wonderful vacation scene by the ocean: a golden beach, toasty warm sand, the pleasant warmth of the sun. Try to feel the ocean breeze, smell the scent of the ocean, and taste the salty water. Imagine foamy white waves breaking against the shore and then retreating to the ocean. You can hear the waves; they come and go…come and go… You are looking at the water, at the distant horizon. You are not sure where the water ends and where the sky begins. You feel good, very good and peaceful. White clouds sail across the blue sky, together with your thoughts, and disappear in the distance. You feel simply wonderful.

The respiration of the ocean becomes one with your breathing. The sound of the breaking waves becomes one with the sound of your heartbeat. You immerse yourself in this place. You are part of this place. You are an ocean of peace. <u>The peace that is inside you right now did not come from the outside. It has always been there. You have it within you at all times.</u> You simply don't realize that it is inside you or you choose not to access it.

In the state of deep peacefulness, you are in touch with your inner sacred space. You can name it sacred space, soul, the subconscious, or inner child. It is multilayered and multidimensional. To keep things simple, I will name it "subconscious" or "inner child." This is a very important place. For most people, reaching a level of higher consciousness can happen only through this place. Finding the way to your super conscious is like finding the key to the reserve of energy, wisdom, inner peace, and healing power that is available to all of us in the universe.

The super conscious has many levels and is multidimensional. You can find different names for it: higher self, collective consciousness, higher consciousness, divine consciousness, higher source of power, universal consciousness, cosmic consciousness, or God. Regardless of which name you choose, regardless of which level you reach, you can reach high enough to have an excellent source of great wisdom and power. From this source, you can draw the power to fortify your health and mental stability. How can you do it? One time-tested method is Visualization.

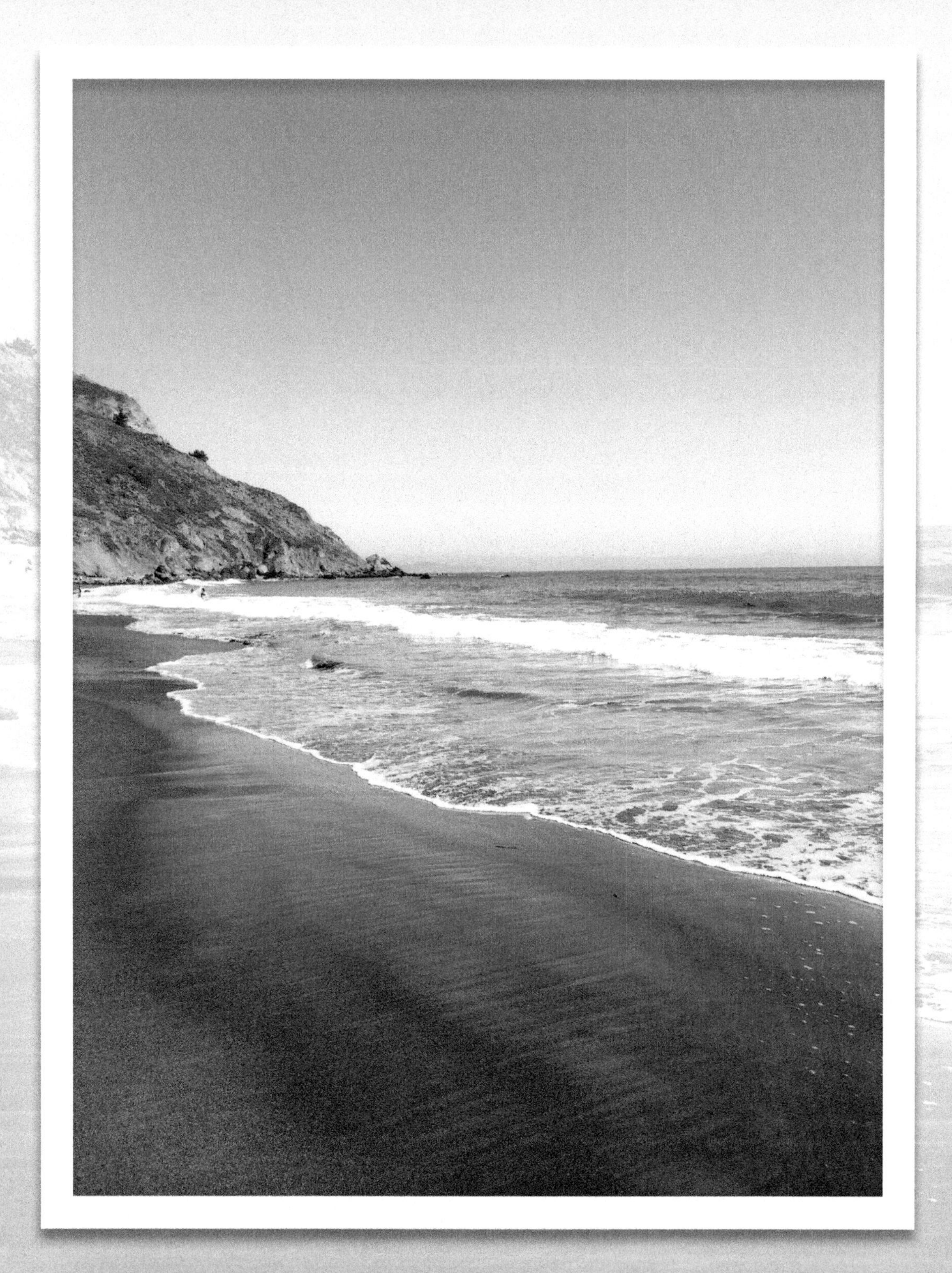

VISUALIZATION

Visualization should be employed after relaxation, meditation, or prayer. That is when your mind is calm, and you are in touch with your subconscious. The subconscious is the bridge that connects your consciousness to the super consciousness. Some people have a direct connection between consciousness and super consciousness. But most of us can reach this higher source of power and make our visualizations effective only through the subconscious. The subconscious does not distinguish between past, present, and future. Everything happens "now," in real time; for this reason, during visualization, use only the present tense. By working with your subconscious, you can expand your perception of the world and better understand yourself and others. This is also the place where our experiences and memories are stored. Sometimes our early experiences from childhood have a big impact on our adult life. You may have phobias, fears, or emotional scars that can be traced to early childhood experiences stored in the subconscious.

I would like to give an example from my own life. For years, I had suffered from claustrophobia. I recently spoke with an aunt who told me a story about my childhood. While my parents were at work, my grandmother cared for me. She loved me greatly, but she was very ill, and was not able to chase after a very active two-year old. So, I was kept in a large wooden box, which was used for making dough for bread. When I heard this story, it was an "aha!" moment – I discovered the origin of my claustrophobia. I followed the practice of the Polynesian Kahunas; I worked with my inner child. In my meditation, I visualized myself as a toddler inside this wooden box. I saw fear and hopelessness on the little girl's face. I picked her up, held her, hugged her, kissed her, and told her, "you are OK, you are safe, and I love you very much." I saw her face changing. There was no more fear or tension. She smiled, and said, "I love you too." After this visualization, I was not affected very much by claustrophobia any more. I still don't like small, closed spaces, but it is nothing in comparison to my previous "phobia."

You can work with any issues from your childhood in the same way I did, or differently. Remember that whenever you give your inner child love, a sense of safety, and treat your inner child well, you become healthier.

Sometimes we don't understand why we feel we are not enough, even though we achieve some degree of expertise in a field, we have a job we love, a family, etc. The source of this feeling is deep inside in our childhood. Little children see reality differently than adults. A small, unimportant incident (to an adult) can be very traumatic for a child, and can cause a huge impact in his/her adult life. Lack of confidence, phobias, fears, feelings of insufficiency, guilt, or unworthiness may be traced to a particular childhood experience. You can help yourself, even if you don't know the source of your adult problems. You can simply talk to your inner child. Give your inner child unconditional love, hug him/her, and tell him/her: "You are beautiful, you are good and worthy. You are not alone. You are safe. I love you."

I used visualization for the first time when I was twelve years old, and I did not have any idea what visualization was about. I was hospitalized after an emergency surgery. I had a very high fever, and nothing was working to lower it. I was unconscious and had a vision or hallucination. I am not sure what it was, but it was so vivid and so alive that I remember it in detail even today. I found myself on a beach on the Baltic Sea, which I had visited many times. I knew that the water was very cold, and I never liked the first moment of getting into the cold water. But this time it was a pleasure. I felt the cold water around me cooling my hot skin and giving a lovely release of the heat and the pain, washing them out. I was swimming, free and happy, and really enjoyed this cold water. It was absolutely wonderful. Then I found myself in bed – with no fever. I did not understand what happened, but the result was fabulous. My experience illustrates beautifully how visualization can be used to alter a state of the body in reality. When you experience a high fever, imagine yourself slowly getting into the water at your favorite lake, sea, or ocean. Imagine that you are swimming. You feel cold water surrounding your burning body, refreshing you and bringing relief. With this type of visualization, you can really lower your temperature.

If you have health problems, imagine a visit with your doctor. The doctor examines you, looks at test results, and smiles, "everything is fine." This visualization creates an impulse, sufficient enough for your subconscious, in connection with higher consciousness, to start a chain of reactions leading to health improvement.

If you suffer from an infection, imagine a battlefield; you are mobilizing an army and you are the general. It is not important what sort of army you choose. You can imagine professional trained soldiers with modern equipment, or a ragtag army. It is not important, as long as you win the war. This kind of visualization will mobilize your immune system to fight the germs that are causing the infection.

If any part of your body does not work as it should, visualize mending it. You don't necessarily need to know how the part works. Through visualization, you can repair it in any way you like. If you are a car mechanic, listen to the engine. Tighten a screw, change a broken part, and make it work, as it should. If you are a cleaning person, sweep, polish, and throw all the garbage away. Tidy everything, and let it be as good as new. If you are a doctor, use a laser, scalpel, cut it out, do a transplant.

How can you speed up the healing of broken bones? Imagine that you are looking at the fracture, see the breakage lines. Visualize very bright white light radiating up and down along broken bone. Watch the broken bones merging together. They are strong again. They are already healthy, and you can move around.

Visualization is especially helpful to cancer patients. Even though science has made tremendous progress in treating cancers, the side effects of chemotherapy, and radiation therapy are grueling and sometimes very hard to endure. Chemotherapy and radiation damage young, quickly-multiplying cells, which means mostly cancer cells, but also bone marrow, blood cells, mucous membranes, skin, hair, and nails. Targeted therapies and immunotherapies are more precise in fighting various types of cancer, and can spare more serious adverse effects on surrounding healthy tissues. Still, the side effects have not been eliminated. How can you support yourself using visualization while receiving cancer treatment?

Imagine cancer cells are targets for chemical particles and radiation. You can protect the healthy cells and organs with special covers. In your imagination you can build walls, fences – anything you can think of that might be effective. Imagine cancer cells dying, and you immediately sweep that post cancer garbage away, flush it out, throw it away.

You can also choose a "peaceful" route. The cancer cells are rebels. Imagine surrounding them with great love, telling them they are a part of a whole, which can't function without them. You make them realize how important they are for the body. If they refuse to cooperate, the body that supports them will die, and they will die with it. They can only survive if they work together again and operate as an integral part of the body. Now the rebellious cells are ready to return to normality. Visualization of this kind enhances your body's ability to self-regulate and regenerate.

If the above images don't work for you, think about encapsulating the tumor. Close the violent cells in the capsule, like in a jail, isolate them from the rest of the body. Close and squeeze them in that small box, so they don't interfere with your everyday life. It works very well in the case of prostate cancer and different kinds of tumors.

Prior to your cancer treatment, you receive medications to prevent the side effects of chemotherapy. Nevertheless, despite the medications, many patients suffer from nausea, vomiting, diarrhea or constipation, rash, mucositis, neuropathy, and many other unpleasant symptoms. How can you help yourself in that situation? Obviously, you should be sure to discuss your symptoms with your doctor. Perhaps your medications need to be adjusted or the course of the treatment needs to be changed. In addition to any help from your doctor, you can apply relaxation and visualization to improve your well-being and eliminate or decrease the side effects of chemotherapy.

As always, start with regular, deep breaths, loosen up your muscles, and relax your mind. Close your eyes, and imagine yourself in your favorite place. Let us say that is the beach. You are lying on warm sand. You look at the water, and see the color of the water and the sky. The waves come, climb the shore, and return to the ocean. You hear the sound of the waves crashing against the shore. You can feel the wind on your skin, and can smell the scent of the ocean. You are feeling good, very good and peaceful. Imagine your stomach, and fill it with a wonderful green elixir of peacefulness, calm it down. Let the golden sunshine penetrate your liver and kidneys. Fill your belly with warm orange liquid. It is very special, magic liquid that repairs and regenerates everything… You feel better.

During chemotherapy your bone marrow can be damaged or blocked, and you can encounter various complications. Bone marrow is where the blood cells are produced. A low level of hemoglobin and red blood cells means anemia, tiredness, and lack of energy. A low level of white blood cells means that you can catch all kinds of infections very easily. Germs that are harmless to a healthy person, can cause a serious threat. Even a family member who has a minor cold can cause you a serious pneumonia. If the number of platelets goes down, bleeding can occur for hardly any reason or no reason at all. When the level of hemoglobin or platelets is too low, you might need a blood transfusion. If your white blood cells are too low, you might receive an injection that gives the bone marrow a boost to produce more white blood cells. These treatments are very effective, but your health will improve much faster if you support yourself with visualization.

After chemotherapy, your bone marrow looks as if a tornado went through it. You need to rebuild your bone marrow. This is where visualization can help greatly. Imagine a newly built factory manufacturing beautiful, healthy, and high quality blood cells. Next, imagine visiting a doctor. In your imagination see the doctor looking at your test results, being surprised, and saying "Your body is coping tremendously, the test results are excellent." See yourself with your family and friends, laughing and joking. See yourself as happy and healthy as you can be.

I have given you some specific examples, but you can visualize whatever you need, utilizing images you find helpful. You have access to a source of power, and your body can use it to achieve better health. If you need to, read this chapter again, and begin using visualization according to your own needs. Good luck!

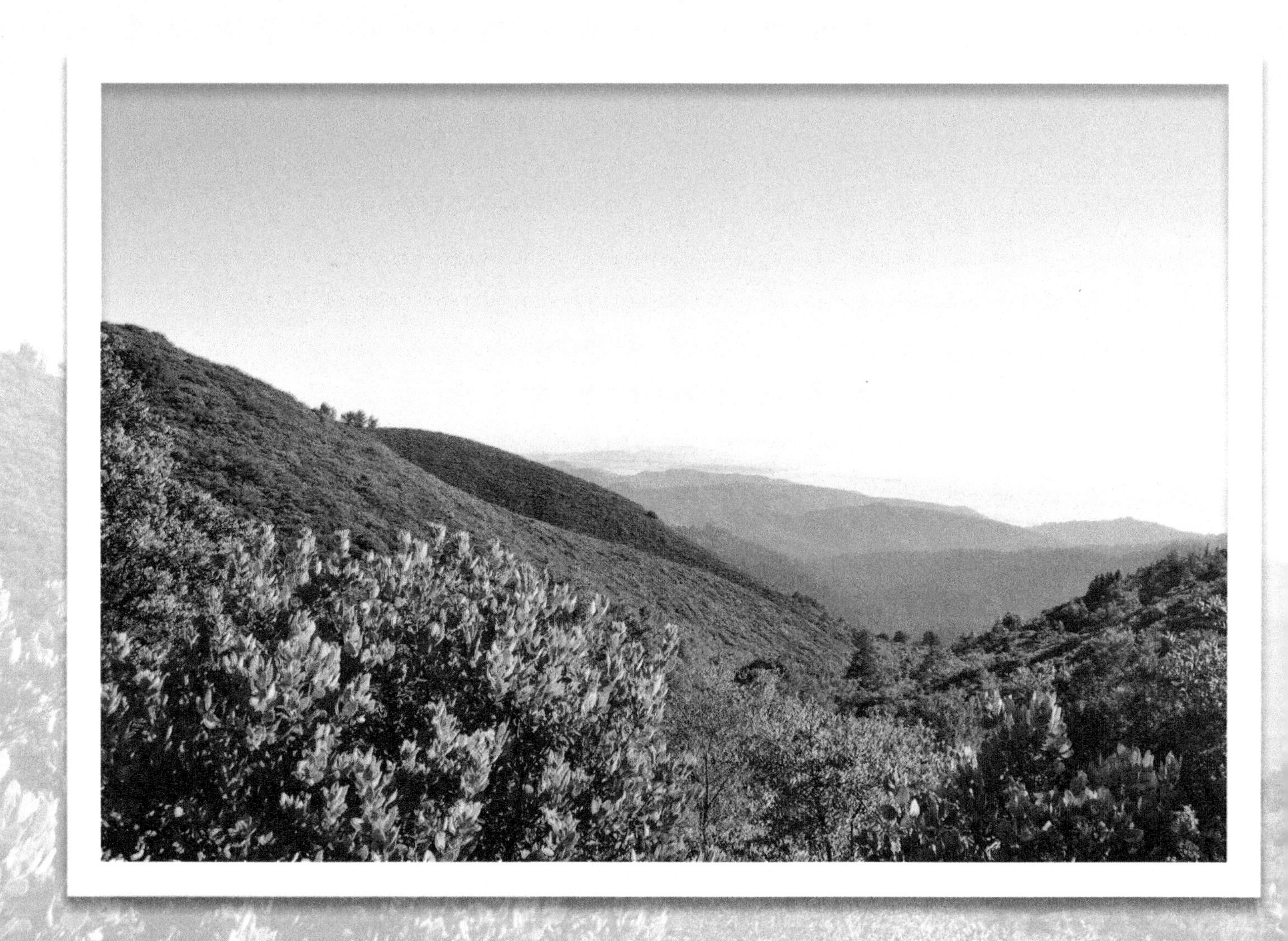

ENERGY POWER OF YOUR BODY

You already know the tremendous power of your thoughts, emotions, and imagination. Now it is time to explore another type of your own power – energy power.

The source of energy for our planet is the Sun. Plants are able to use solar energy to produce organic food from nonorganic components. This food is the main source of vital energy for animals. Plants and animals are the source of energy for humans. We eat, digest, and absorb various nutritional substances. These are distributed throughout the body by the blood. Some of them are used as building materials, some as supplies for the future, and some are transformed into energy in the body's cells. For this "transformation" to occur, we need oxygen. That is why breathing is very important.

Certain parts of our body need more energy than others. Energy flows inside the body on various levels: between cells, tissues, organs, and body parts. Some of that energy travels in the blood, some along the nerves, and the majority flows in special energetic channels that eastern cultures call **meridians**. All the channels (meridians) contain centers for exchanging energy between various levels inside the body and with the outside world. These centers for exchange and regulation of energy flow are called **chakras**.

The study of energy flow in and around the body originated thousands of years ago, most probably in India. Chakra in Sanskrit means "a wheel." Some people see chakras as turning wheels of light, as multifaceted flowers, or as whirlpools with tunnels opening at the front and back of the body.

You do not need to know all the complicated theories about meridians and chakras. All these theories agree that chakras are centers for regulating energy flow in human body and energy exchange with the world.

Meridians are like rivers of energy flowing through your body. Stress-related muscle tension or mechanical obstructions block energy flow. On one side of this "block" there is a flood of energy, on the other side there is a drought – too much energy on one side, too little on the other. Both sides manifest themselves with pain or malfunction of the organs.

The most common cause of meridian blockage is **stress**. Stress is an indispensable part of life. In life-threatening situations, stress can give you the strength to survive through the "fight or flight" response. However, long-term stress usually becomes the source of illness.

Since you cannot eliminate stress from your life entirely, you need to learn to live with it, minimize its effects, and maybe even learn to use it in a positive way. If you are completely honest with yourself, you can find the source of your stress. Usually, having analyzed it deeply, impartially, and without emotions, you will find a solution to a stress-related problem. Sometimes you will discover that you need to change your life style, slow your pace, or allow yourself to rest. On other occasions, you may remind yourself of abandoned responsibilities, small or major dishonesty, or of dreams that were never realized. Listen to yourself; it is your private lesson. Do not judge yourself. Be gentle with yourself. Just learn your lesson. Stress does not necessarily have to make your life more difficult. It can change your life for the better. However, before that happens, you must correct the existing effects of stress by restoring the proper flow of energy in your body.

Energy blockages can be removed by well-functioning chakras, especially if we support them with relaxation or specific exercises, such as yoga, tai-chi, qigong, or Tibetan exercises. You might also opt to use massage, acupuncture, acupressure, reflexology, bioenergy therapy, or EFT/Tapping. They all work, so choose the one that works for you and reap the benefits.

You can also apply the techniques that I am going to introduce now. They are easy and simple, even if they seem a bit abstract in the beginning. They are based on clearing and energizing the seven most important chakras in the main energy channel running along your spine. Every chakra works on a different frequency, has a different color, a different vibration, and regulates different endocrine glands, nerve plexuses, and organs. Let us have a closer look at them:

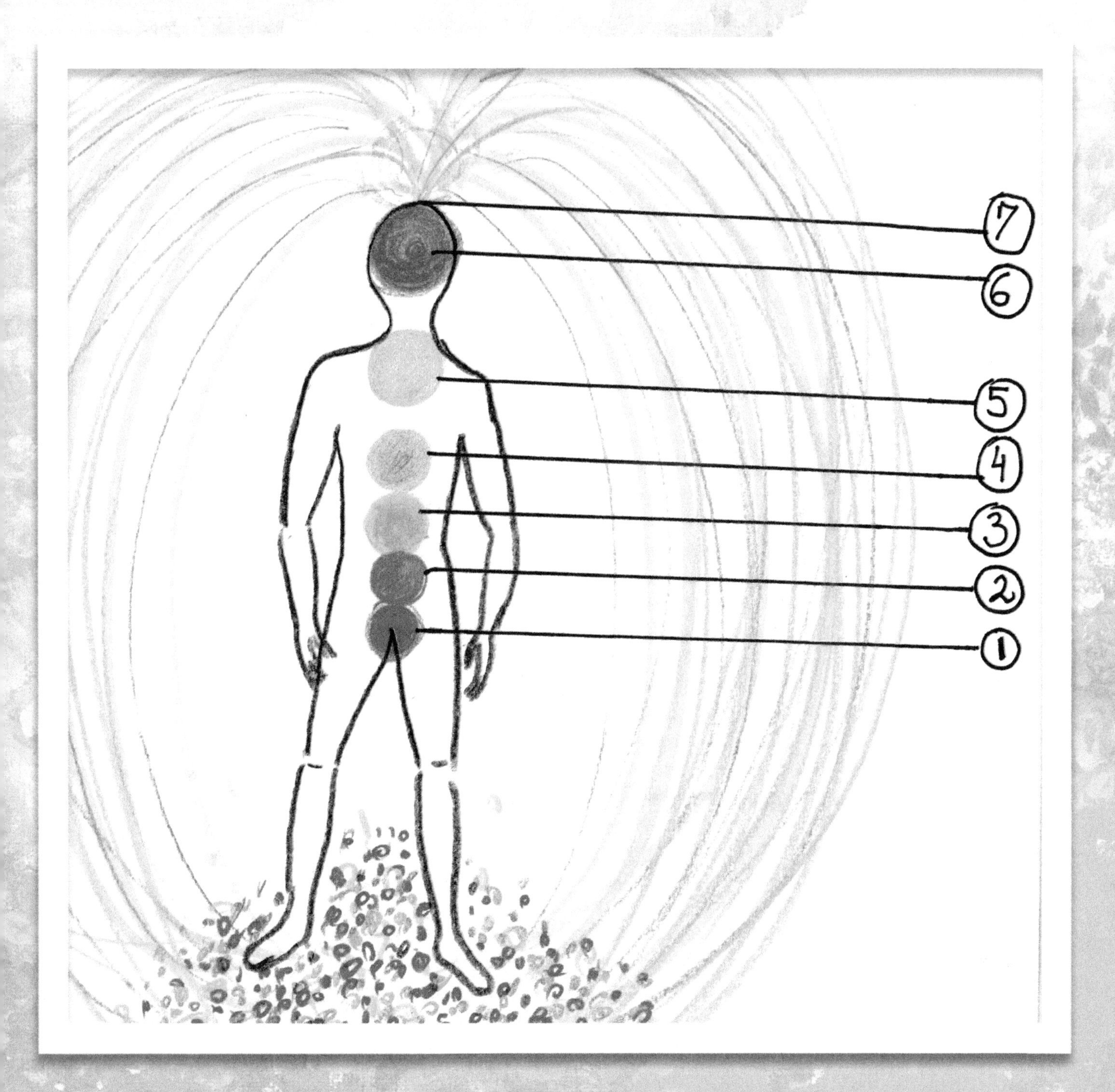
7
6
5
4
3
2
1

The First Chakra (Base/Root Chakra)
Color: Red
Location: Base of the spinal cord
Function: Responsible for vital life energy, the energy that powers the turbines of physical life and supports self-preservation. It controls the musculoskeletal system, partly the reproductive system, regulates the process of cellular growth, and the creation of blood cells.

The Second Chakra (Sacral/Spleen Chakra)
Color: Orange
Location: Between the pubic bone and the navel
Function: It partly controls the reproductive organs, the bladder, the spleen, and part of the digestive system. Affects the quality of blood, immunity, sexual well-being, and creativity.

The Third Chakra (Solar Plexus/Personal Power Chakra)
Color: Yellow
Location: A little bit above the navel
Function: It is related to the liver, gall bladder, pancreas, kidneys, partly the stomach and intestines. This is the chakra through which most people exchange energy with outside world. Negative emotions seriously disturb its work. This chakra influences your self-esteem.

The Fourth Chakra (Heart Chakra)
Color: Green
Location: In the middle of your chest
Function: Controls breathing and affects the heart, thymus, partly the lungs and stomach. It is the home of higher emotions, love relationships, and self-acceptance.

The Fifth Chakra (Throat/Thyroid Chakra)
Color: Blue
Location: Base of the neck
Function: Responsible for the thyroid and parathyroid glands, lymphatic system, trachea, larynx, throat, and partly the lungs. This is the home of empathy and compassion. When this chakra is not functioning well, you might have problems with self-expression.

The Sixth Chakra (Third Eye Chakra)
Color: Indigo
Location: Between the eyebrows
Function: Controls the pineal gland, coordinates all the other main chakras and the neuro-hormonal system. Responsible for clear thinking, enhanced perception, intuition, and communication with the subconscious.

The Seventh Chakra (Crown Chakra)
Color: White (the synthesis of all colors)
Location: Top of the head
Function: It is the chakra of enlightenment and the center of pure divine consciousness. It controls the brain.

I am now going to suggest and describe three simple techniques you can use for restoring the correct work of the chakras and proper energy flow. These techniques are based on refueling the internal and external energy fields of the body, using the energy that surrounds us.

This might sound strange, but you are surrounded by an ocean of energy that you can use. This energy has various names: ether, prana, mana, chi, universal creative force, universal life energy, universal energy, cosmic energy, life force energy, and life energy field. Your material body is like static energy, more or less dense. Specific energy states keep transforming one into another and influence each other. The energy is in constant motion, and the energy equilibrium is always dynamic. If you are interested in the science of energy, there are some interesting books you can read on quantum physics: Albert Einstein's theory of relativity, the works of Nikola Tesla, Wlodzimierz Sedlak, or Albert Szent-Gyorgyi.

To make things easier, I will describe in simple terms the human energetic body, and its connection with cosmic energy. Your body is surrounded by a seven-layer energy field, with each layer related to one of seven chakras. Any disorders in this energetic field are manifested by changes in the material body, and vice versa – changes in the physical body can cause disturbances in the surrounding energy field. By clearing, reinforcing, and restoring the energy field, and by correcting the energy flows inside and around your body, you can regain strength and health.

If the above explanation helps you understand the work with bioenergy- excellent. If not, don't worry. In fact, we fail to understand the nature of many things, but we still use them, because they are helpful. Just think, how many people truly understand the nature of electricity? Regardless, we all use it. You do not necessarily need to understand the actual process that takes place when you imagine refueling your energetic system. The important thing is that by using your imagination, you are able to initiate these processes for your benefit.

Technique # 1

This technique aims at replenishing old, stagnant energy in the chakras with new, fresh energy. As always, start with breathing exercises, then loosen all your muscles, relax, and quiet your mind. After that, work with your chakras separately, one by one, using the proper color. You will fill each chakra and the surrounding areas with the color that is associated with that chakra.

The first chakra

Imagine a vivid red color, like that of a ripe apple or a beautiful red rose. Imagine the bottom of your belly infused with this color. If you can see it when you close your eyes, excellent. Exchange the old, stagnant color with the bright, beautiful crimson of a red rose. If you can't imagine it or can't see the color, do not worry. Simply say "I am exchanging the old, faded energy for a wonderful, bright, flaming red."

The second chakra

The color is bright orange. Fill your intestines with orange light. Just like with the first chakra imagine or verbalize exchanging the old color for a new, bright orange. Now your intestines are starting to work better. Your immune system protects your body more efficiently.

The third chakra

Let bright golden-yellow sun rays penetrate the area surrounding your navel. Let them caress, warm, and bring to full life all the neighboring organs, including the kidneys, liver, gall bladder, and pancreas.

The fourth chakra

The color for this chakra is green. Fill the middle of your chest (stomach, heart) with the fresh, bright green of spring grass.

The fifth chakra

Imagine a blue sky on a sunny summer day. The air is clear, translucent, and pure blue. You inhale that blue, fill your throat, and lungs. It is invigorating and refreshing. You feel so much better.

The sixth chakra

Imagine the purple-red, indigo color of the setting sun, bringing calm and peace. Fill your head with that color and with the peace and calm that it brings.

The seventh chakra

Now imagine that having passed along the spine through the main chakras all the colors get combined together and there is a white waterfall of energy erupting from the top of your head, falling to your feet, and creating a protective energy field around your body. This energy then refracts back into the base colors, and re-circulates through your body. You are surrounded by a white, opalescent cocoon, reflecting all the colors of the rainbow. It is safe and quiet inside this cocoon.

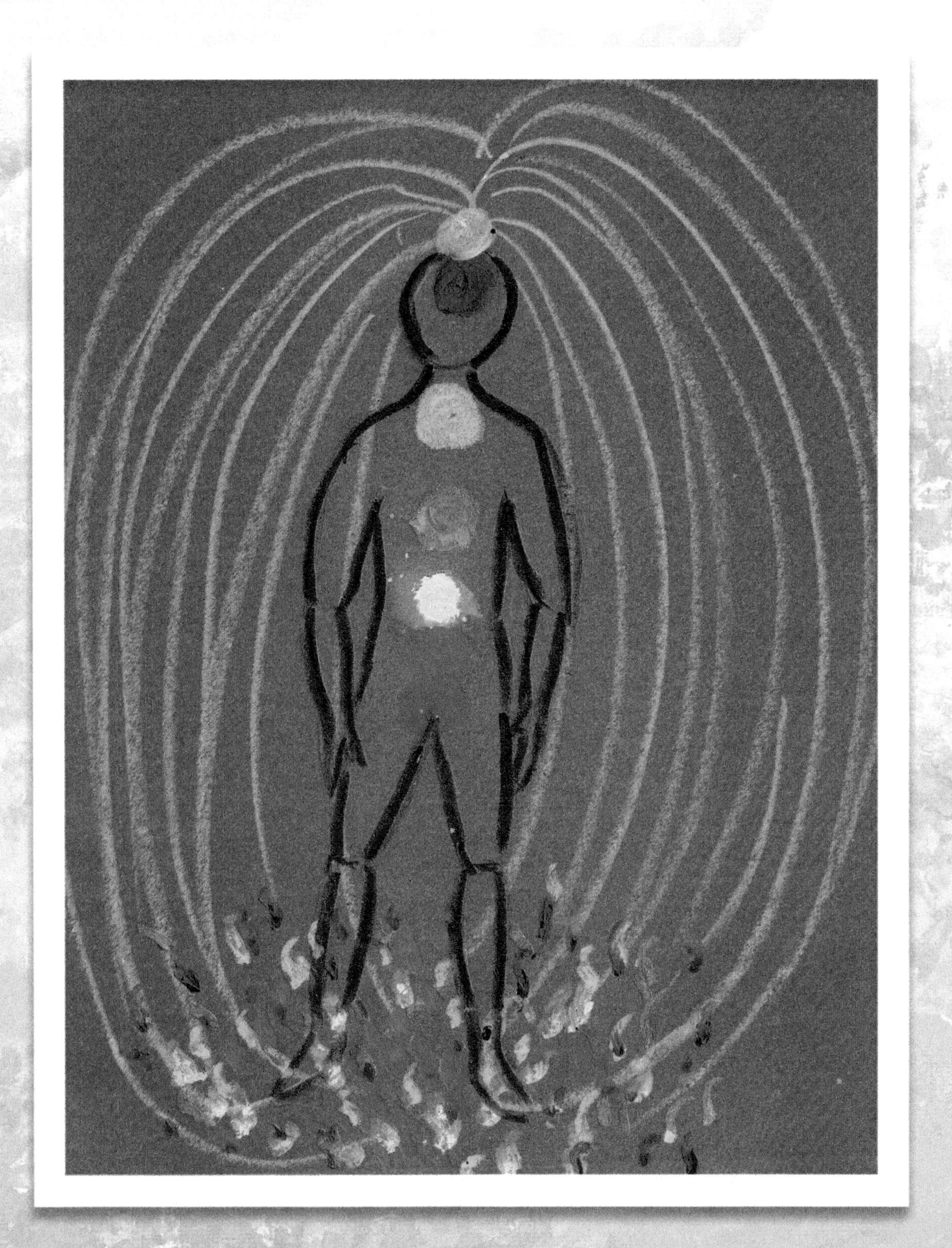

Technique # 2

This technique helps you infuse your body with fresh energy through the chakras. It requires that you use your hands – fingers and palms - as detectors and transmitters of that energy. They are very powerful tools for exchanging energy with the surrounding world and with other beings (in fact, your palms are chakras, too!). To begin to feel the bioenergy field with your hands, I recommend the following exercises:

Exercise 1:

Sit down, relax, with your hands on your thighs, palms up. Observe your hands, feel them. Then elevate your hands up a little bit and position them with the fingers of one hand opposite those of the other hand, separated by about 12 inches. Draw your fingers near, and then pull them apart. Move your hands slowly back and forth until you find a distance when you feel something. It can be a very delicate tingling, heat, cold, pulsation, pushing, or pulling. When you look at the space between your fingers, you can see energy flowing. It is like a very delicate smoke or gauzy light. If you don't see anything, don't worry. After practice, your perception will expand and you will be able to see the energy flow.

Exercise 2:

You can also use your palms to feel the flow of energy. Elevate your hands and position your palms about 12 inches apart. Move your hands slowly, back and forth, until you notice some feeling. Again, it can be tingling, heat, cold, pulsation, pushing, or pulling. You can have these feelings on right or left hand, or on both. It is very individual and whatever you feel, it is good. Notice this distance, notice your feeling, and remember it. From this distance, you can always find a connection with your own bioenergy field, or with the energy field of others.

Use the following drawings to guide you in the above exercises.

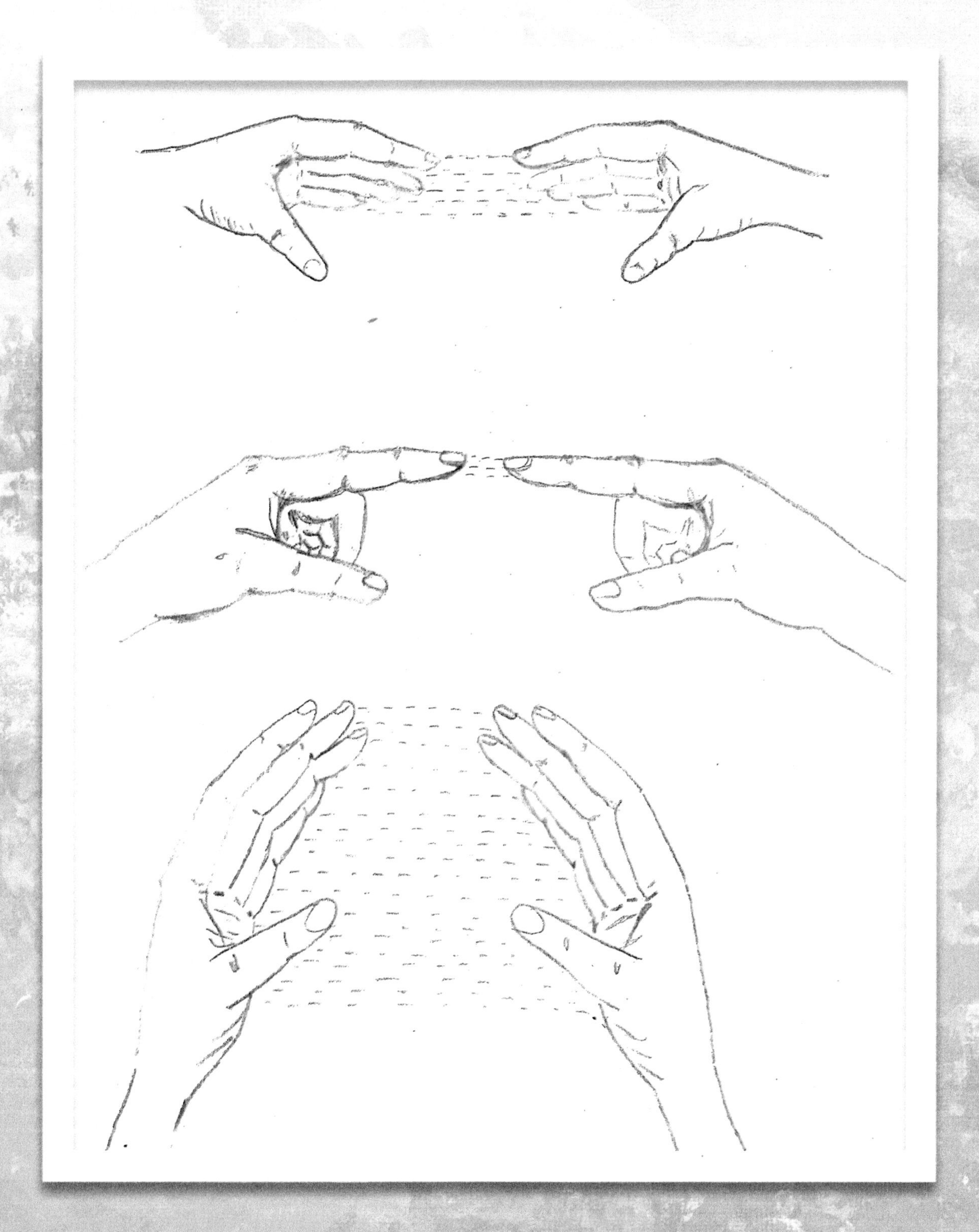

Once you feel the sensation of energy flowing through your fingers and palms, you are ready to use the technique of infusing fresh energy into your body through your chakras. If you don't feel anything even after the above exercises, don't worry. Not everyone will feel the energy, but it doesn't mean that it's not there or isn't flowing. Your intention is the most important factor in this technique. Remember that energy follows your thoughts. Wherever your attention and your thoughts are going, the energy is going there too.

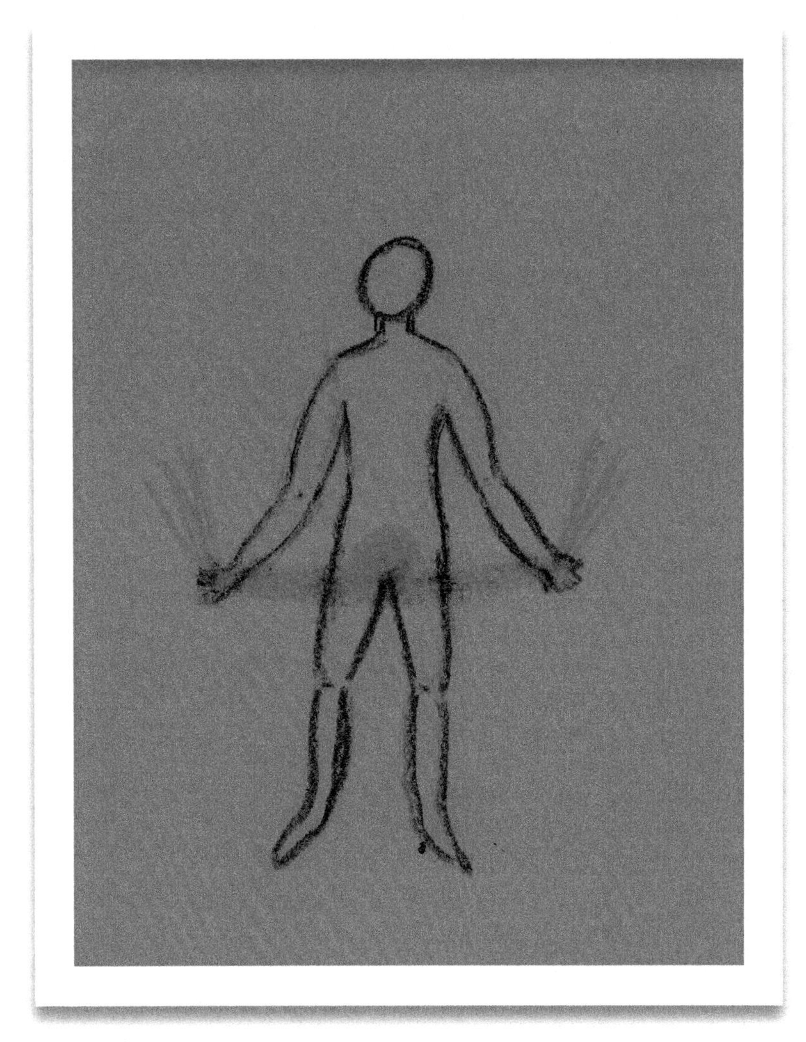

Let's begin infusing each chakra, one by one, from the first one to the seventh. Stand with your legs slightly apart and your hands loose at your side. Turn your palms so that they are facing upwards, lift them sideways just a little bit, and position them on the level of the **base chakra**. Imagine your hands are channeling a wonderful, life giving energy from the air into the first chakra. You can add the color. The red light fills the bottom of your pelvis, clears, refreshes, and refuels the chakra. The first chakra is connected to the first energy layer around your body – fill it with bright red. You may feel the warmth, vibration, pulsation or tingling in your hands and body. If you do not feel anything, do not worry. Your imagination has already kick-started the re-energizing process, so carry on.

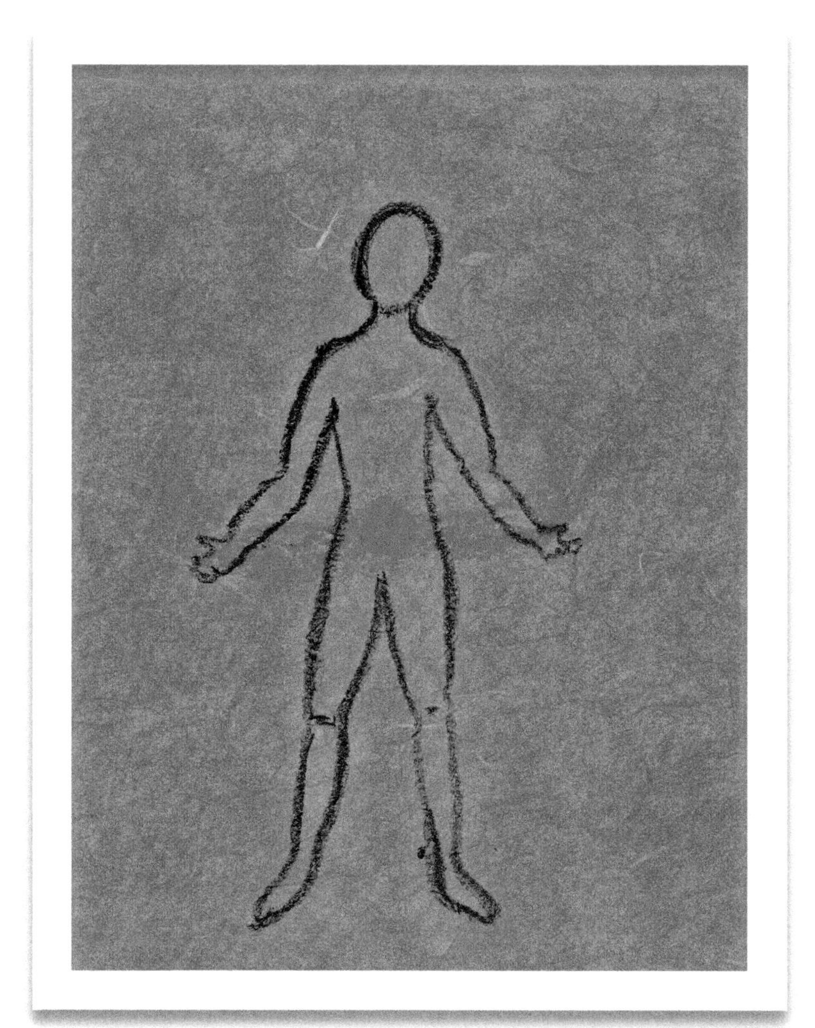

Now lift your hands to the level of the **second chakra**. Imagine a stream of orange light flowing through your hands and supporting the sacral chakra and the second energy layer. Exchange the washed-out color for the lively orange of a ripe orange fruit.

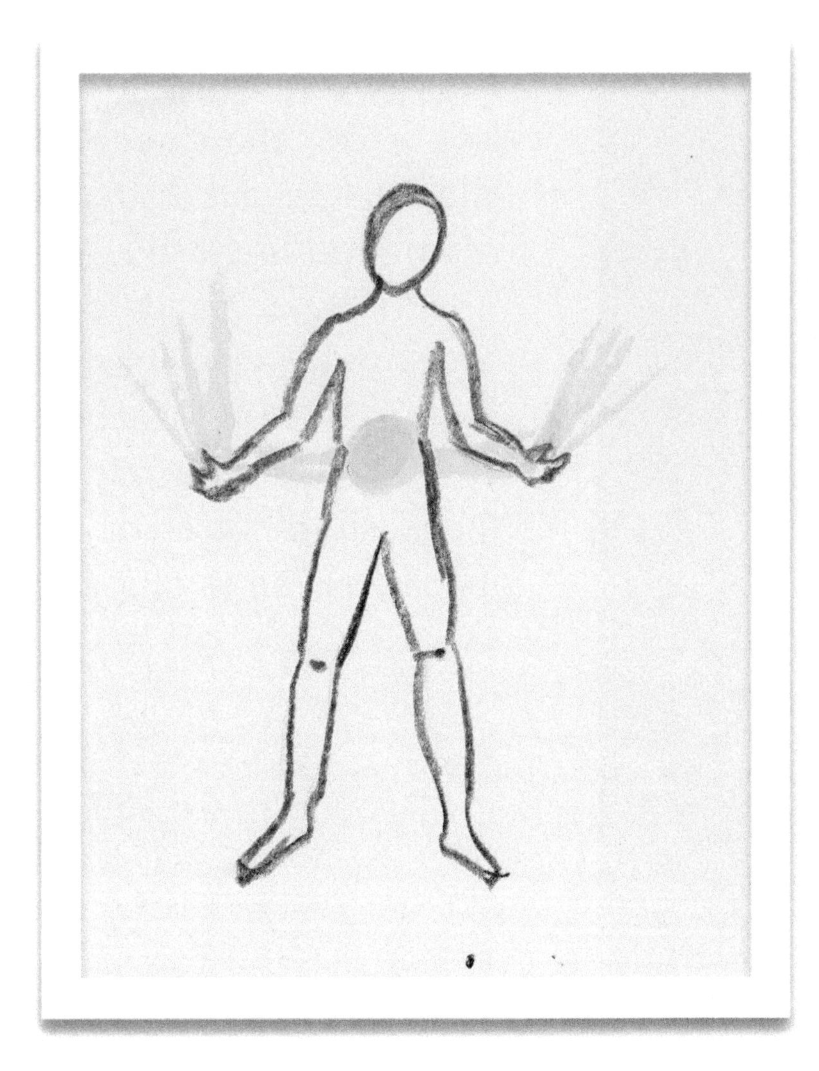

For the **third chakra**, elevate your palms to the level of your navel and imagine the bright yellow of the sun. Take in the yellow prana from the air and channel it into the solar plexus chakra and to the third energy layer around your body.

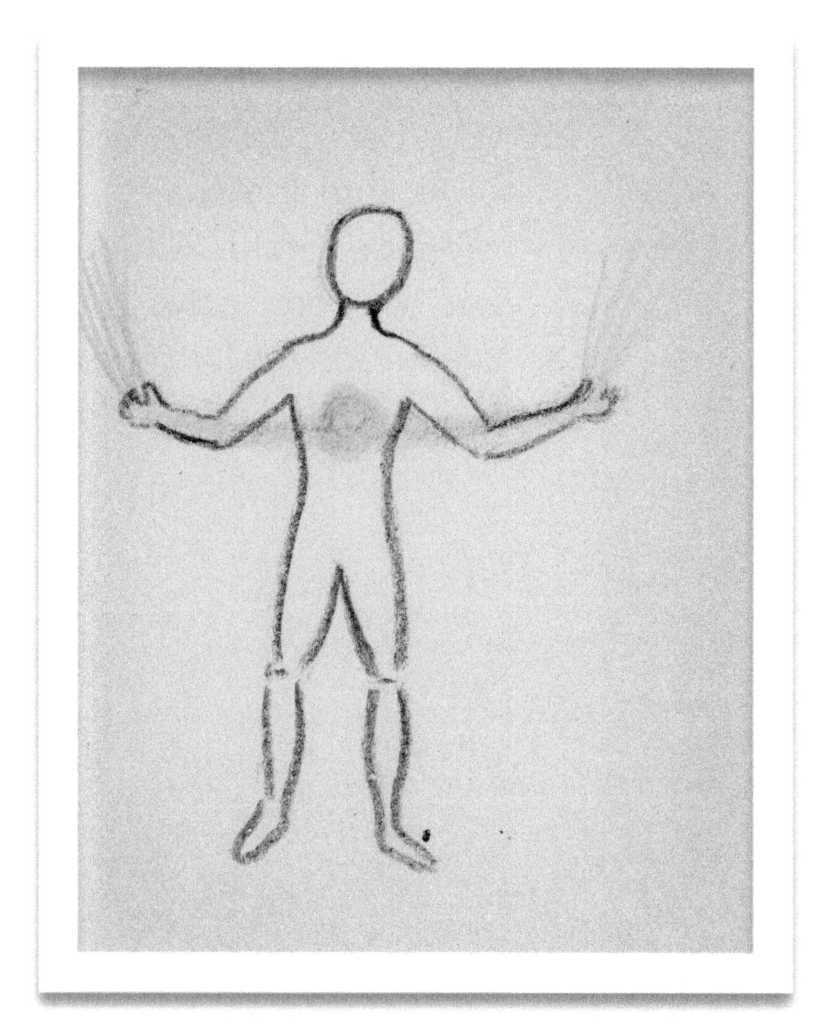

Now, you clear and re-fuel the **fourth chakra** and fourth energy layer by inviting the green prana through your hands elevated up to the chest level.

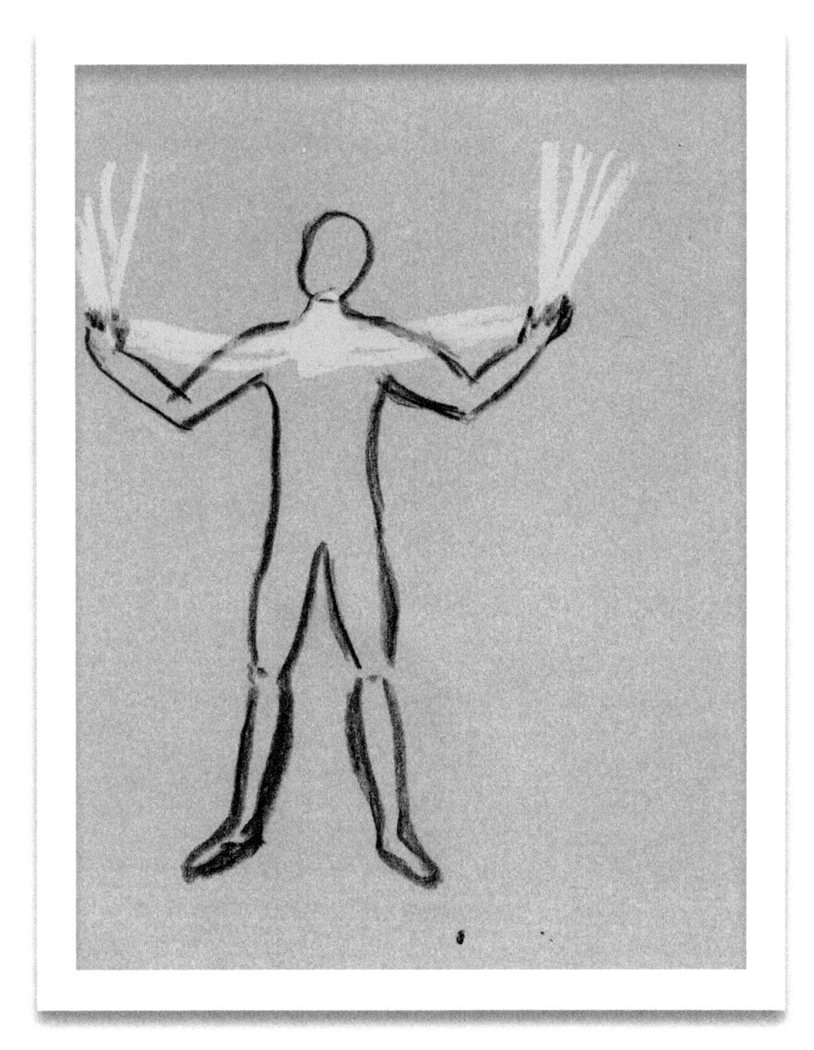

For the **fifth chakra**, raise your palms to the height of your neck. Visualize the sky-blue prana. Cleanse and re-energize the throat chakra and the fifth energy layer with the blue light.

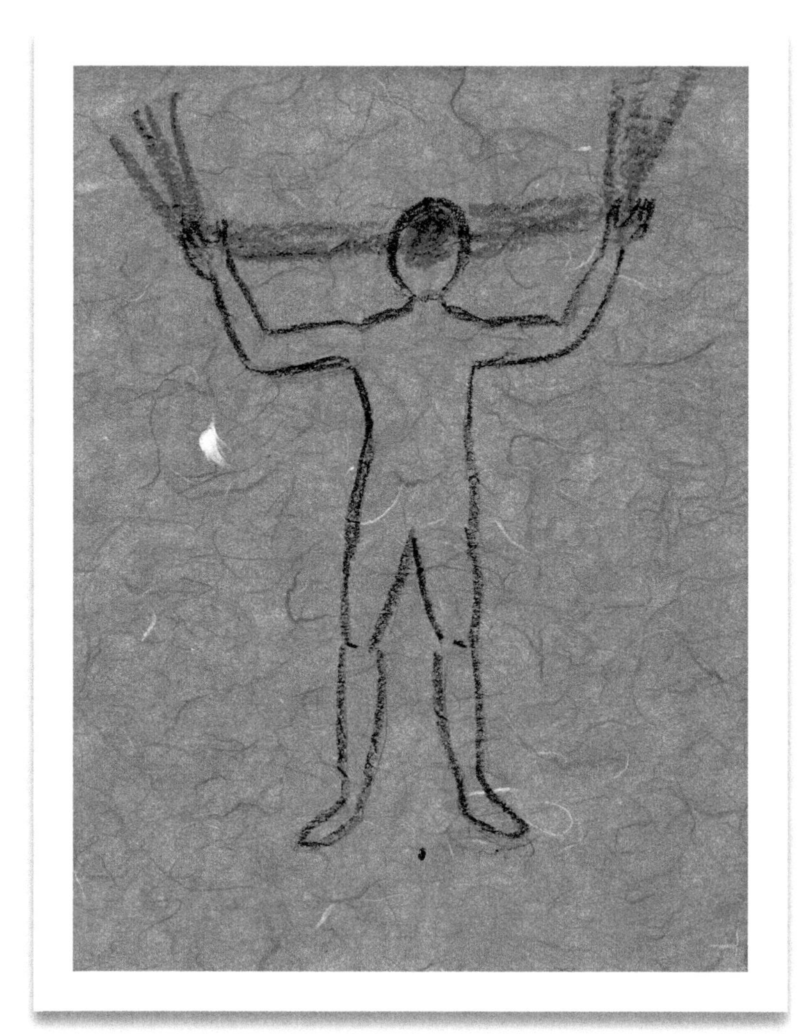

For the **sixth chakra**, arms are held wide-open, palms level with your forehead. You are now attracting the indigo-colored prana. Clear your head and the sixth energy layer around your body and fill them with fresh, luminous energy and indigo light.

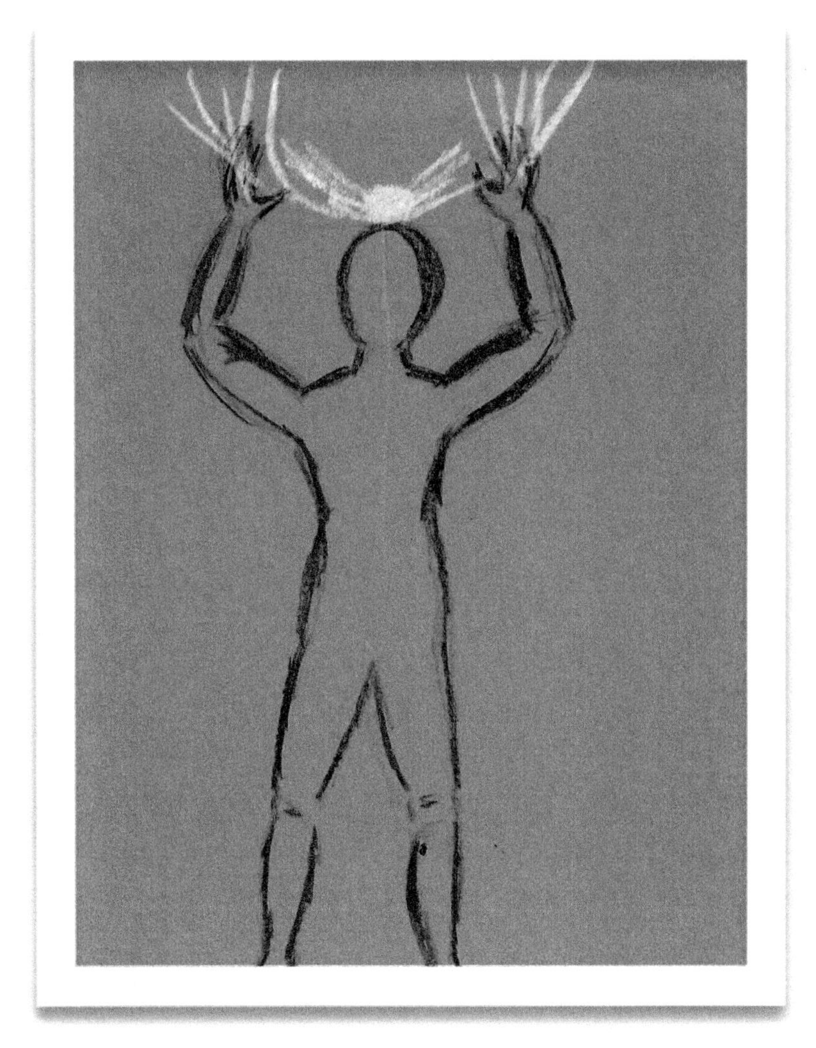

The **seventh, crown chakra** is on top of your head. Lift your hands and hold them up, as if in the act of blessing. Imagine a silver-white stream of energy flowing into your palms, giving light, surrounding, and protecting you. You are now a ball of rainbow light. You are glowing. You are an energetic pump. Let the energy flow from the first to the seventh chakra; pump it through all the chakras, one by one. Flush out the pools of stagnant energy, wash them out, and replace them with clear, fresh, shining energy.

Using the power of this new energy, you can remove all energy blockages. You can add some sound to this exercise. Each chakra vibrates differently, operates on a different frequency, and synchronizes with a different sound. The seven notes of the major scale correspond to the seven chakras in harmony. As follows: C is typical for the first chakra, D for second chakra, E for the third, F for the fourth, G for the fifth, A for the sixth, and B for the seventh. Adding these tones will assist in moving energy blocks.

The exercise I just described should make you will feel better; after completing it you should be more energetic and lively. You can repeat it as often as you want and whenever you want – in the meadow, in the forest, on the beach, or at home. If you are unable to stand up, do it while sitting or lying down, but do try to keep your spine as straight as possible.

Technique # 3

In this technique, you use your hands for channeling energy to improve the work of any malfunctioning body part. Let us say you have problems with your stomach. First you have to clean the stomach area of stale, stagnant energy. Put one of your hands above your stomach, palm down, and then imagine you are "throwing away" sick energy. In order to reinforce the action, make repeated movements to "throw away" this bad energy. Now, raise your hands to stomach level, with palms up. Imagine that you are collecting wonderful green prana. Fill your palms with this pure green healing energy, and apply it to your stomach. Let the healing energy flow to the stomach.

Here is another variation of this technique:
Position your one hand above the place or organ, which needs improvement, palm down. Use the other hand like an antenna/radar to find the frequency which is in harmony with what you need. Just move this hand around, circle up and down; until you will feel the flow of energy between your hands, like a wave … That is it. Fill yourself with healing energy.

You can use the above-described techniques to support every part of your body and every organ.

Technique # 4

I found this technique through my practice. It will enable you to balance your chakras and to achieve balance between the physical and spiritual aspects of your life. This is a very powerful form of healing.

Sit down comfortably on a chair with your spine as straight as possible and with your feet flat on the ground. Begin to breathe, relaxing your muscles and your mind. Elevate one arm above the head with the palm up, and the other direct towards your feet with the palm down. You may feel tingling or other sensations on your palms. Imagine that your hands are like antennas and you are collecting energy from higher sources in Heaven and from the Earth. Energy from Mother Earth supplies our physical functions. Energy from higher sources nourishes our spiritual aspects.

Now, move your hands. Move one hand to the level of your crown chakra (#7) and the other hand on the level of your basic chakra (root chakra, #1), with palms turned toward your body. Feel the energy flow from hand to hand. If you do not feel anything, imagine that you are sending strong energy beams from the first chakra up to the seventh chakra. If this is difficult to feel, try reversing the direction and sending strong energy beams from the seventh chakra down to the first chakra. Some people have a stronger physical aspect to their life (a stronger connection to the Earth), while others have a stronger connection to the spiritual aspects of their life, which is why your choice of the direction in which you send the energy might make a difference. If you still don't feel anything, that's ok, too. A lack of sensation doesn't mean that the energy is not flowing. Simply keep going through the exercise.

There may be a blockage between the first and seventh chakras. You can use your source of stronger energy (Earth or Spirit) to flush out the main energetic channel in your body. When you feel the energy flow between your hands, you know that your main channel is clear. Play with this energy for a while. Observe it, contemplate it, and enjoy it.

Move your hands to the position of the sixth and second chakras with palms turned toward your body. Feel the flow of energy. In the beginning, you may feel only weak impulses; observe how these impulses grow. Feel the waves of energy going from one hand to the other, back and forth.

The next position will be over the fifth chakra (thyroid, at the base of the neck), and over the third chakra (the solar plexus, just above the navel). Feel the energy flowing from one hand to the other.

Now put both of your hands on the middle of your chest, on the heart chakra. This is the most important and beautiful moment; the meeting of Heaven and Earth in your heart. This is your sacred place in your heart. Here you are with Mother Earth, and your heavenly Father. You have all the power offered by the Earth and Heaven. From here, everything is possible.

When you feel discomfort, tension, or pain in some part of your body, send to this place the energy from your heart, with the intention to restore normality and well-being. Do this until the discomfort, tension, or pain subsides.

Contemplate for a moment this power that you have, and then allow your energy to flow up to the crown chakra, and out of your body, like a fountain of light surrounding your body, giving you extra protection, strengthening your energy field, and repairing all disturbances inside of it.

This is the most powerful method of balancing chakras that I know. Give it a try, and you will feel much better.

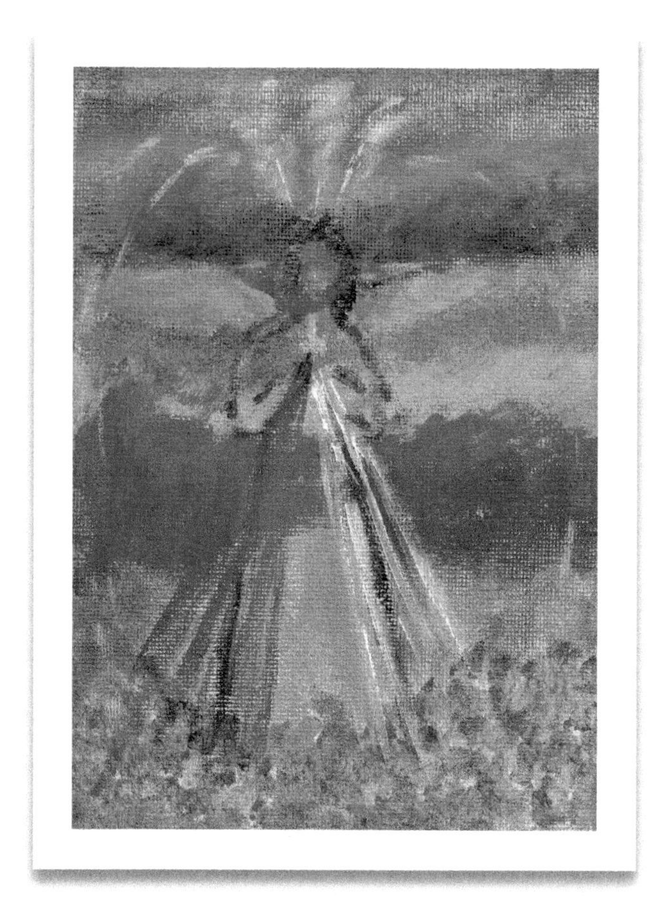

Your body has a tremendous ability for self-regulation and healing. Your job is to find the key to open the door to the reserves of energy and power to heal every aspect of your life on physical, emotional, mental, and spiritual levels. You can work with your energy field to correct your physical problems, or you can work with your emotions to correct your health on the physical level. You can combine energy work with work on your emotions and get great results. That's what EFT or Tapping does. Let see how it works.

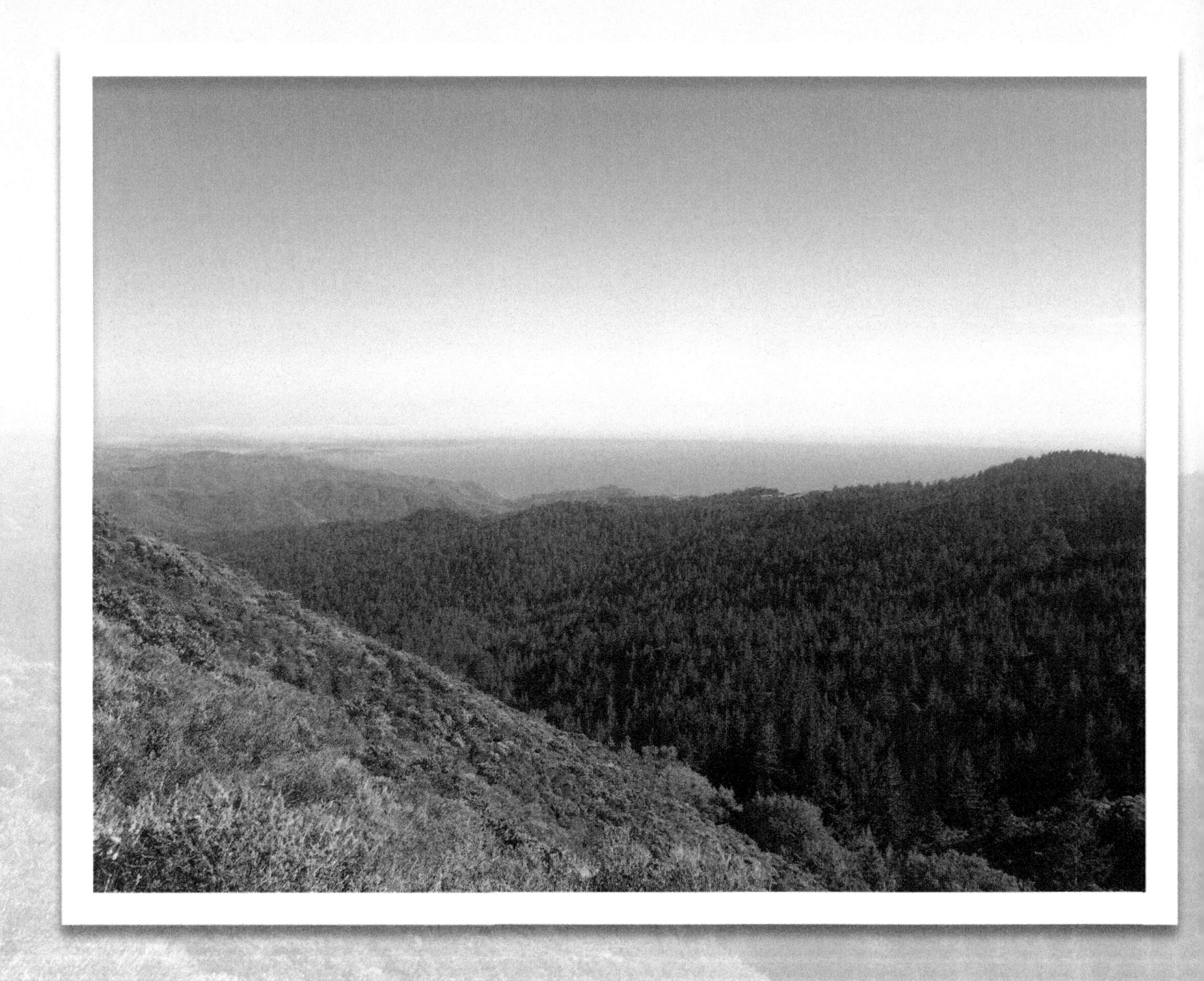

TAPPING OR EFT: EMOTIONAL FREEDOM TECHNIQUE

Dr. Roger Callahan, a psychologist, who was also interested in acupuncture, started what is now known as EFT about 30 years ago. He was working with a woman who had a severe water phobia. She was afraid of the ocean, swimming pools, bathtubs, and even the rain. After one year of traditional therapies, she was able to sit on the edge of a swimming pool, and put her feet in the water. During one session, she revealed that thinking about water caused terrible feelings in her stomach.

It was Dr. Callahan's "ah-hah!" moment. He asked her to tap on the end of the stomach meridian, which is located on the cheek bones below the eyes, hoping this would help alleviate her stomach discomfort. It helped her not only with the stomach, but also with her water phobia. That was the beginning of what is now known as EFT (Emotional Freedom Technique).

Meridian Tapping, or EFT is a stress relief technique that combines modern psychology with some of the elements of acupuncture. We tap with our fingertips on appropriate acupuncture points while verbalizing our problem. This way we are able to access the storage of long-term memory and emotions in the amygdala, the oldest part of brain. The amygdala reacts on the basis of the "fight or flight" response. During this type of response, numerous chemicals and hormones are released into the bloodstream preparing us to be stronger fighters or faster runners. This can save our life in dangerous situations. However, even for minor stress, the amygdala reacts as if a "fight or flight" response is required. Prolonged (long-term) stress, even minor, means continuous high level of chemicals and hormones released by the amygdala. These can have a negative impact on our health. In fact, this causes more than 90% of all our health problems. Tapping is a technique that can release old and new stress created in our bodies through the "fight or flight" response.

Sometimes we do not know or do not want to remember the source of the stress related to a current problem. My friend had a traumatic experience from her childhood; she was horribly abused by her father, and now she has serious health problems. She tried to work with the positive thinking technique without success. I tried to work with her through forgiveness and healing her inner child. This also did not work. The memory of her childhood was still too painful to touch. In her situation, tapping was the ideal solution. During tapping she talked about her current problems, current feelings, and current emotions.

Amazingly, her old traumatic wounds were healed, and her health has significantly improved.

Most cancer patients experience fear, anxiety, or even panic attacks at some point during their therapy. Fear and anxiety are not your friends. They can strip you of energy and suppress your immune system, which is not good, especially when you struggle with cancer. When you experience anxiety or a panic attack, rationalizations usually don't work. You need some sort of an "emergency kit." For my patients in this critical moment the best emergency technique is tapping or EFT.

The very first time I used tapping was at work. I was caring for a patient who had a panic attack during a blood transfusion. I stayed with the patient, while the nurse in charge called the doctor and another nurse ran to the hospital pharmacy to get the medication ordered by the doctor. All of this took some time. I was alone with a patient who was agitated and emotionally unstable. She wanted to pull her IV out. In my imagination, I could foresee the consequences of such a move: her blood splattered on the walls and the ceiling. I had to do something immediately. Instead of giving the patient explanations and rational reasons for why she should not pull out her IV, I asked her to tap with me to relieve her anxiety. She did not know anything about tapping, and I did not have time for any explanations, so I asked her to copy my movements and repeat phrases after me. The patient was surprised enough to follow my unusual proposition. After a few minutes of tapping, we were laughing and the patient was perfectly fine.

I use tapping a lot to ease patients' journey through chemotherapy. It might be a technique that seems a little strange for you, but I encourage you to try it. It really works. Through tapping, we can release any old and new stress, and improve our health.

So, how to do tapping?

- Choose one problem that bothers you right now.
- Rate the intensity of your problem on a scale from 0 to 10 (0 = no stress, 10 = intolerable stress).
- Create a set-up statement, which is accurate for you in this moment. Verbalize your problem, but also include a statement about self-acceptance, which is critical to the success of the tapping process. One example is: "Even though I am anxious, I deeply and completely accept myself."
- Start tapping on the "karate chop" point (as illustrated in the drawing), while repeating the set-up statement three times.
- Tap on the specific points on your face and upper body, while mentioning the problem, the associated thoughts, feelings, emotions, and beliefs related to this problem. Be honest.

- Once your negative experiences, emotions, and beliefs have been processed, you are ready to be positive again in a deep, authentic, and powerful way. Now you can truly accept yourself.
- You are ready to say, "It is time to change. I am free from anxiety. I feel good and safe."
- Once you have finished tapping, take a deep breath and rate the intensity of your issue using the 0-10 scale to check your progress.
- Repeat as necessary to get the relief that you desire, or move on to a different, more pressing issue.
- When you are tapping, try to be very specific. For example, "I am anxious" is not very specific. Say: "I am anxious, because I received a bad diagnosis, I have cancer."

Let's do a tapping exercise to clear up anxiety related to a diagnosis of cancer. We will be tapping on various points throughout the body, starting with the "karate chop" spot and moving on to some others.

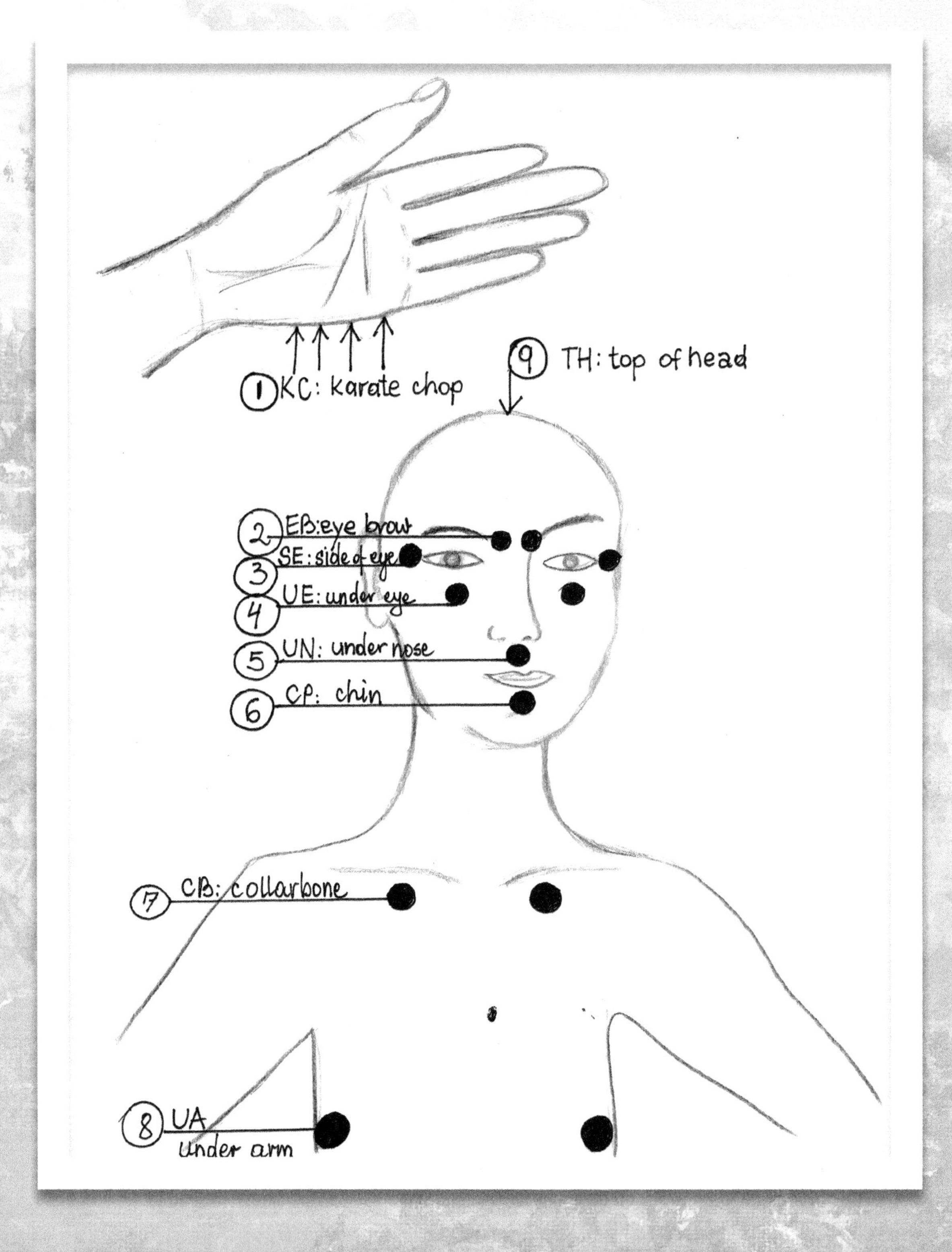

1 KC: karate chop
9 TH: top of head
2 EB: eye brow
SE: side of eye
3
UE: under eye
4
5 UN: under nose
6 CP: chin
7 CB: collarbone
8 UA
under arm

Point # 1 – External edge of your hand, or the "Karate Chop" point
Tap on the "Karate Chop" point on your hand and repeat these set-up statements:

- "Even though I am diagnosed with cancer, I deeply and completely accept myself."
- "Even though I am scared to death when I think about me and my family's future, I fully and completely accept myself."
- "Even though I am so anxious, I still love myself, I respect myself, and fully and completely accept myself."

Point # 2 – Eyebrow
"This anxiety"

Point # 3 – Side of eye
"It is really scary."

Point # 4 – Under the eye/cheek bone
"I hate this diagnosis."

Point # 5 – Under the nose
"What can I do?"

Point # 6 – Chin
"With this anxiety, I cannot think clearly. I am almost in panic."

Point # 7 – Collarbone
"Why has this happened to me?"

Point # 8 – Under the arm
"Now, everything is upside down in my life."

Point # 9 – Top of head
"I have a choice to be calm, but I am not quite ready..."

Point #2 – Back to eyebrow
"I do not have any idea how to free myself from anxiety."

Point # 3 – Side of the eye
"Even though I am still anxious about my future, I accept myself."

Point # 4 – Under the eye
"It is safe to let go of the fear and anxiety."

Point # 5 – Under the nose
"I cannot change my diagnosis, but I can change my feeling about it."

Point # 6 – Chin
"The fear and anxiety will not help me at all."

Point # 7 – Collarbone
"It is time to say *'Goodbye'* to anxiety."

Point # 8 – Under the arm
"But, I still feel this tightness in my chest."

Point # 9 – Top of head
"I choose to accept myself anyway."

Point # 2 – Back to eyebrow
"Even though I still feel some anxiety, I know I am safe."

Point # 3 – Side of eye
"I still want to cry, when I think about my diagnosis."

Point # 4 – Under the eye/cheek bone
"It is OK to cry."

Point # 5 – Under the nose
"Even though I am crying, and cannot think clearly, I still respect, and accept myself."

Point # 6 – Chin
"I feel a little lighter now."

Point # 7 – Collarbone
"The doctor told me that I have a chance."

Point # 8 – Under the arm
"I feel that I have a big chance."

Point # 9 – Top of head
"Everything will be OK. I have a plan, support, and help. It is time to be anxiety free. I am strong, and safe."

Take a deep breath. Rate your level of anxiety. If it is not satisfactory, start tapping again until the anxiety is relieved.

This is only one example. You can work this way with all your problems, emotions, and pain. If you want to learn more about this method, I strongly recommend the book "The Tapping Solution" by Nick Ortner, or his website www.tapping solution.com.

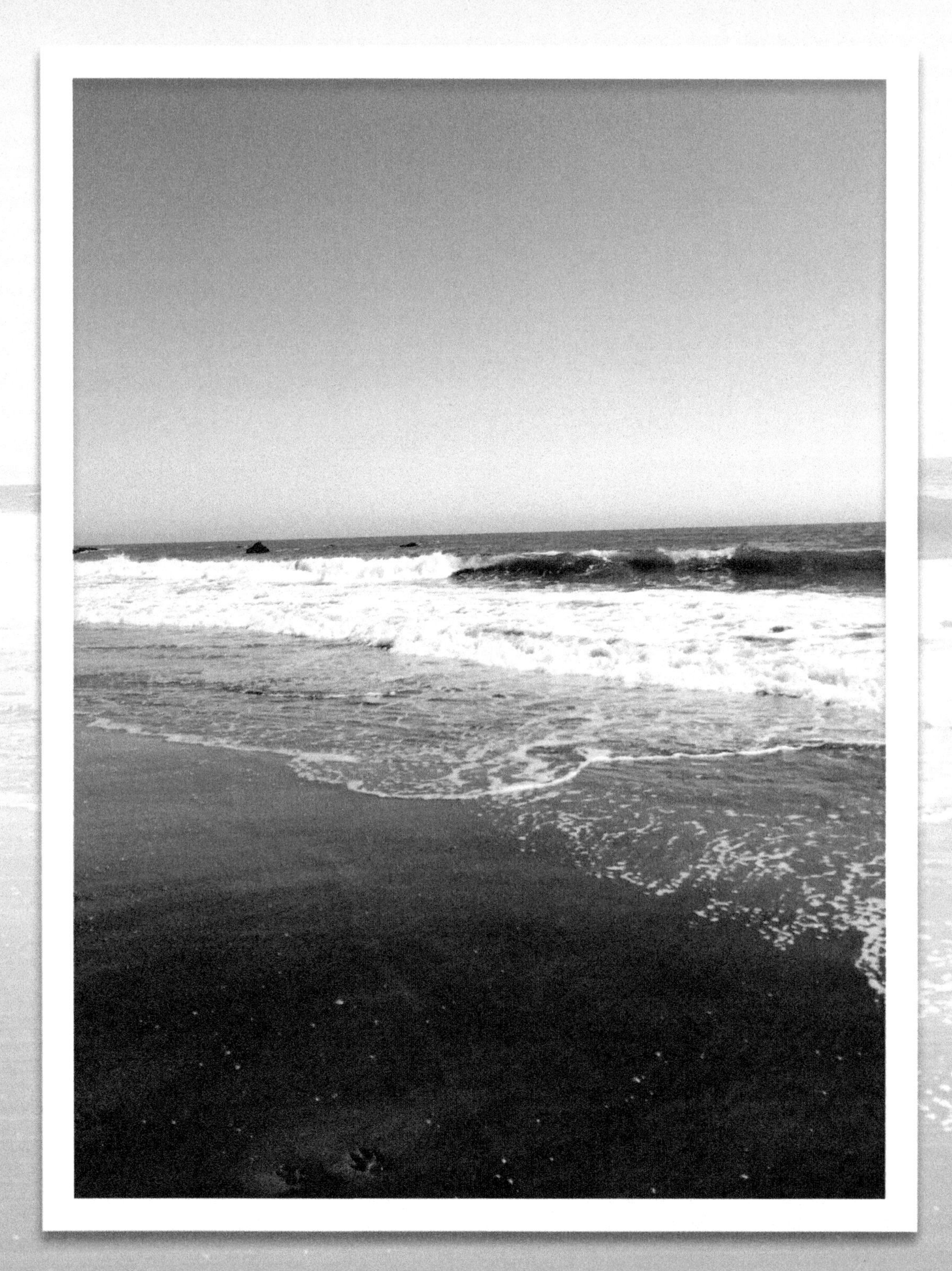

OTHER USEFUL STRATEGIES

If for some reason you cannot start energy work by yourself, you can always ask a professional therapist for help. When you cannot start your car because battery is very low, you ask somebody for a jump start. An energy therapist in any specific field you choose can give you a "jump start" when your personal battery is low, when you feel a lack of energy.

All energy therapies are based on the transfer of life energy, healing energy, from the higher source through the therapist to the recipient. There are many different methods of transferring healing energy and different types of healing: Bioenergy Therapy, Bio-puncture, Therapeutic Touch, Healing Touch, Laying on of Hands, Polarity, Forensic Healing, Chakra Healing, Pranic Healing, Reiki, Matrix Energetics, Quantum Healing, Spiritual Healing, etc. All types of energy therapies are non-invasive. There is no pressure, manual manipulation, or massage to the body. The client remains fully clothed at all times.

I was once giving bioenergy support to a patient of a well-known and very respected oncologist. The patient was receiving chemotherapy at the time. The doctor was surprised how quickly the healing was progressing and how well the patient was feeling during chemotherapy. When the doctor heard about the bioenergy therapy, he was less than thrilled. He was worried it could spoil the great results of his chemotherapy treatment. He thought that if bioenergy was indeed stimulating blood cell production, that it probably also would stimulate cancer cell growth. This may be logical, but is not correct. Bioenergy therapy and other types of energy work restore proper energy flow in the patient's body and improve body function. This improvement of body function includes blood cell production and at the same time enhancement of body's ability to fight cancer. All bioenergy work can be used during chemotherapy for the patient's benefit.

Below is a list of therapies, which can support you during chemotherapy. You can choose one or more that you think can help you.

Prayer

An honest, deep prayer – your personal conversation with God while your soul is at peace – can bring a huge relief from suffering. Prayer lifts the vibrations of your body, enabling access to divine energy, enhancing the healing process, and relieving pain. You can expect similar results when other people are praying for you. You can pray to God, archangels, angels, or to the saints. You can say the rosary or repeat mantras. There are holy words, holy sounds, and holy symbols that can make it possible to get in touch with a higher source of healing energy.

Music

You yourself know best what kind of music can calm you and enlighten your soul. You can also buy professionally recorded relaxation or meditation music. Music has the unique power to open hearts and minds. Different sounds resonate with corresponding chakras by specific vibrations, frequencies, and wave lengths. There are seven chakras. The first corresponds with the sound of "Do," the second with "Re," and so on. Through music you can tune yourself like a musical instrument. Every person has a characteristic style, and everyone can find the right music to bring harmony into his/her energetic system. Some people find Mozart helpful, others Bach, Beethoven, or Chopin, or something from other musical genres. For someone else Tibetan singing bowls might be the most beneficial. Try and you will find something that works for you.

Bio-emanative Brain Linking (known as the BBL, or BSM method)

This method is based on putting hands on the patient's head, above the brain centers that control specific functions of the body parts. Energy emanating from the healer's hands activates those centers to initiate the healing process. Craniosacral therapy does the same job as BBL/BSM by manipulating the bones of the skull with an extremely light touch.

Acupuncture

This is a form of Chinese traditional medicine. It is based on stimulating specific energy channels with special, tiny needles. It is not painful. The needles are disposable, used only one time. It is a safe procedure, but should be done only by certified acupuncturists. Electro-acupuncture is a variation of traditional acupuncture. It is stimulation of specific energy channels with a special electric device.

Acupressure

Acupressure is based on applying pressure to strictly specified points on the human body along the energy channels. Pressing stimulation points opens up the energy channels, releasing energy to disordered parts of your body to help them revert to proper function. Calming points reduce energy activity in responding channels, quieting you and reducing pain.

Reflexology

Reflexology is another type of bodywork that restores energy balance through massage and putting pressure on certain reflex points on your hands and feet. You can have reflexology done professionally. You can also ask a friend or family member to massage your feet, based on instructions from a professional reflexology book.

Chiropractic Therapy

Chiropractic therapy improves alignment of the spine and restores the normal flow of nerve impulses by using spinal manipulation. Chiropractors believe that the spinal cord, as a main line of communication between body and brain, is the key to restoring health.

Massage Therapy

There are more than 100 methods of massage. They use manipulation of the body's soft tissue by hands, forearms, elbows, and sometimes even feet. Massage can reduce muscle tension, enhance general relaxation, improve blood circulation, lymph movement, mobility, digestion function, and help to optimize and maintain health.

Massage is wonderful in general, but it is not for everyone. Ask your doctor if you can use massage therapy, as it is not advisable in certain types of cancer.

Physical Therapy

A physical therapist makes an in-depth professional assessment of an individual patient's needs, and chooses the proper therapy and exercise regimen. The therapist can help you regain fitness, release pain, improve your movement, coordination, and general well-being.

Physical Exercise

Nothing makes the body feel better than a bit of physical activity. You do not need to do complicated, strenuous exercises. In the beginning you may ask your family to assist you. Start by exercising all the joints, one by one. Move your toes, fingers, feet, knees, hips, wrists, elbows, and arms. Move them upward, downward, left, and right if possible. Do circular motions. Bend your spine forward, backward, and twist sideways. Bow and roll like a ball. These simple exercises will improve your blood, lymph, and energy circulation. If you prefer some guidance during your exercise, try to attend a tai-chi, qigong, or a yoga class.

Aromatherapy

Aromatherapy uses essential oils to relieve symptoms. You can use essential oils for inhalation, applied to the skin, or in a drink. For example, you can inhale Eucalyptus oil to relieve a cough, a problem with breathing, or for an infection of the respiratory tract. You can use Mint essential oil for relief of nausea/vomiting by inhalation, in a drink, or by applying it to the inner side of your wrist. For neuropathy – Mint, Myrrh, or Frankincense can be helpful. You can ask an herbalist to advise which essential oils will benefit you and how to use them. Before using any oil, do an allergy test. Put one drop of the essential oil on the inner side of your forearm. Observe this spot for half an hour. If you do not see any changes on your skin, you can use this oil. If you observe any swelling, redness, rash, or if it is itching, you should not use this oil because you may have an allergic reaction to it. Since there are so many essential oils, you can try a different one.

Herbal Therapies

Herbs are very potent plants, and should be used with caution. You can always drink mint tea for upset stomach, but if you want to take some herbs or herbal supplements to treat your disease, consult with your doctor, pharmacist, or herbalist. Herbs should be selected carefully, depending on your disease, condition, medications, and diet.

Homeopathic Treatment

Homeopathic remedies are made from herbs, animal products, and minerals. Homeopathy is based on the theory that a person's vital force is sensitive to sub-molecular homeopathic medicines. Homeopathic remedies are prepared for an individual client's needs. Certain remedies are repeatedly diluted and shaken, until an extremely small amount remains. A micro dose resonates with a person's body and energy field better than a big dose.

The medical community has become increasingly interested in utilizing unconventional therapies to support a patient's recovery of health. This is very good news for patients, but remember: even the best doctor in cooperation with the most gifted healer will not be able to heal you, if you yourself do not take an active part in this process. Your body has tremendous ability of self-regulation and healing. Your job is to find the key to open the door to your own reserves of energy and power to improve your health on physical, emotional, mental, and spiritual levels.

I think you are already on the right path to finding your own way, inner balance, serenity, and strength to successfully support your body throughout the healing process.

With all my heart, I wish you ALL THE BEST!

BIBLIOGRAPHY

1. Alke Harald D. "Leczenie czakramow energia Kundalini", Studio Astropsychologii, Bialystok 2006.
2. Allgeier Kurt "Cudowni uzdrowiciele", Iskry, Warszawa 1993
3. Bartlett Richard, D.C, N.D. "The Physics of Miracles," Atria, New York 2010
4. Bartlett Richard, D.C., N.D. "Matrix Energetics", Atria, New York 2007
5. Barnett Libby, Chambers Maggie, Davison Susan, "Reiki. Leczenie energia", LIMBUS, Bydgoszcz 1997
6. Blawatska Helena P. "Doktryna tajemna", Interart-Tedar, Warszawa 1995
7. Blawatska Helena,P. "Klucz do teozofii", Interart-Tedar, Warszawa 1996.
8. Bott Victor, M.D. "Spiritual Science and Art of Healing. Rudolf Steiner's Anthroposophical medicine", Amber, Warszawa 1995
9. Brennan Barbara Ann "Light Emerging", Bantam Books, New York 1993
10. Brennan Barbara Ann "Hands of Light", Bantam Books, New York 1993
11. Budzynski Stefan, "Bioenergoterapia-Tajemnice uzdrawiajacej energii" Gadam, Warszawa 1991

12. Byrne Rhonda "The Secret" Atria Books, New York 2006
13. Byrne Rhonda "The Power" Atria Books New York 2010
14. Chopra Deepak, M.D. "Quantum Healing", Bantam, New York 1989
15. Chopra Deepak, M.D. "Perfect Health", Harmony Books, 1993
16. Chopra Deepak, M.D. "God. A story of Revelation" Harper Collins Publisher 2012
17. Copelan Rachel "Hipnoza, klucz do umyslu", Limbus, Bydgoszcz 1994
18. Cranston Ruth "The Miracle of Lourdes", Mc Graw-Hill Book Company, Inc. New York 1955
19. Dalai Lama "Meditations to Transform the Mind", Snow Lion Publication, Ithaca, New York 1999.
20. Dalai Lama "Healing Anger", Snow Lion Publications 1999
21. Dale Cyndi "The Subtle Body. The Encyclopedia of Your Energetic Anatomy" Sounds True Inc. Boulder 2009
22. Decker Georgia M. "An Introduction to Complementary Alternative Therapies", Oncology Nursing Press, Inc. Pittsburg, PA 1999
23. Dixon Todd, "Moc uzdrawiania- Tajemnica sily, ktoralLeczy", Limbus, Bydgoszcz 1995
24. Dr. Dyer Wayne, W. "Change Your Thoughts – Change Your Life", Hay House, New York 2007

25. Dr. Dyer Wayne, W. "The Power of Intention", Hay House, New York 2014
26. Dr. Dyer Wayne, W. "I Can See Clearly Now", Hay House, Inc. New York 2014
27. Eden Donna "Energy Medicine", Penguin Group Inc, New York 2008
28. Ferguson Elaine R. M.D. "Super Healing", Health Communications, Inc. 2013
29. Gordon Richard "Quantum Touch. The Power to Heal", North Atlantic Books, Berkeley CA 2006
30. Hay Louise "The Power Is Within You" Hay House, Inc. New York 1991
31. Hay Louise "You Can Heal Your Life" Hay House, Inc. New York 2004
32. Hall Nicola "Reflexology in a Nutshell", Element Books Limited, Shaftesbury, Dorset 1997
33. Hewitt William W. "Hipnoza i autohipnoza" Medium, Warszawa 1999
34. Hover-Kramer Dorothea "Healing Touch" Sounds True, Boulder, Colorado 2011
35. Jarmey Chris, Tindall Jon "Akupresura w codziennych dolegliwosciach", Delta W-Z, Warszawa
36. Joy Jonsson Melissa "M-Joy Practically Speaking" M-Joy of Being, Inc. Encinitas, CA 2013

37. Joy Jonsson Mellissa "Little Book of Big Potentials" Heart-Field Productions Inc. Seatle, WA 2015
38. Kelder Peter "Zrodlo wiecznej mlodosci", Kleks, Bielsko Biala 1997
39. Klimuszko Andrzej, Czeslaw "Moje widzenie swiata", Novum, Warszawa 1989
40. Knaster Mirka "Discovering the Body's Wisdom", Bantam Book, New York 1996
41. Kornfield Jack "Meditation for Beginners", Sounds true, Boulder CO 2008
42. Krieger Dolores, Ph.D. R.N. "The Therapeutic Touch" Simon& Schuster, New York 1992
43. Lane Deforia, Rob Wilkins "Music as Medicine", Zondervan Publishing House, Grand Rapids, Michigan 1994
44. Laskow Leonard M.D. "Healing with Love", Wholeness Press, Mill Valley CA 1992
45. Lewandowski Piotr "Samoleczenie metoda B.S.M", Aries, Warszawa 1996
46. Long Freedom Max "Magia cudow", Medium, Warszawa 1995
47. Loyd Alexander, Johnson Ben "The Healing Code", Grand Central Publishing, New York 2010
48. Melchizedek Drunvalo "Zycie w przestrzeni serca", Centrum, Warszawa 2006.

49. Melchizedek Dunvalo "The Ancient Secret of the Flower of Life", Light Technology Publishing, Flagstaff, AZ 2000
50. Minich Deanna M. Ph.D., C.N. "Quantum Healing", Conari Press, San Francisco, CA 2011
51. Ortner Nick "The Tapping Solution", Hay house, Inc. New York 2013
52. Perry Wayne"Sound Medicine", The Career Press, Inc. Franklin Lakes, NJ. 2007
53. Piotrowicz Kazimierz "Leczenie przeplywem informacji", ZPH Piokal, Chrzanow 1999
54. Pomorski Marian "Wizualizacja sposob na zdrowie i pomyslnosc",MARPO, Kielce1996
55. Powell Artur E. "Cialo eteryczne", Interart Dartex, Warszawa 1995
56. Powell Artur E. "Cialo astralne", Interart Dartex, Warszawa 1995
57. Powell Artur E. "Cialo mentalne", Interart Dartex, Warszawa 1995
58. Powell Artur E. "Cialo przyczynowe" Interart Dartex, Warszawa 1995
59. Powell Tag I Judith "Wahadelko narzedzie podswiadomosci", Medium, Warszawa 1997
60. Prinser Tari "Yoga for Cancer", Healing Arts Press, Rochester, Vermont 2014

61. Rankin Lissa, M.D. "Mind Over Medicine", Hay House Inc. New York 2013
62. Rodenbeck Christina "Meditation to Go", Octopus Publishing Group Ltd, Great Britain 2008
63. Rossi Ernest, Lawrence "The Psychobiology of Mind-Body Healing",W.W.Norton and Company, Inc. New york 1986
64. Rossman Martin L. "Guided Imagery for Self-healing" H J Kramer/New World Library California 20000
65. Sedlak Wlodzimierz "Bioelektronika", Warszawa 1984
66. Silva Jose, Miele Philip "Samokontrola umyslu metoda Silvy" RAVI, Lodz 1994
67. Silva Jose, Stone RobertB. "Samouzdrawianie metoda Silvy", Neptun, Warszawa 1993
68. Sha Zhi Gang Dr., "Power Healing", Harper Collins Publishers Inc., New York 2002
69. Sherwood Keith "The Art of Spiritual Healing", Llewellyn Publications, St. Paul MN 1985
70. Skarbek Jacek "Reiki, Klucz do serca", Studio EMKA, Warszawa 1997
71. Sogjal Rinpocze "Tybetanska ksiega zycia i umierania" Wydawnictwo EM, Warszawa 1995
72. Steiner Rudolf "Spiritual Science and Art of Healing", Healing Arts Press, Rochester, Vermont1984

73. Stengler Mark, N.D. "The Natural Physician's Healing Therapies", Rentice Hall Press 2001
74. Sui Choa Kok, "Praniczne uzdrawianie kolorami", PWN, Warszawa 1993
75. Sui Choa Kok, "Psychoterapia praniczna", PWN, Warszawa 199
76. Sui Choa Kok, Uzdrawianie energia kolorow", Medium, Warszawa 1994
77. Ulman Ryszard Roman, "ABC bioenergoterapii" PWN, Warszawa 1990
78. Ulman Ryszard Roman, "Wstep do bioterapii", Atea, Warszawa 1999
79. Ulman Ryszard Roman, "Swietlisty czlowiek", ATEA, Warszawa 2002
80. Virtue Doreen, "Chakra Clearing", Hay house, Inc. New York 1998
81. Virtue Doreen, "Earth Angels", Hay house, INC. New York 2002
82. Webster Richard, "Creative visualization for beginners", Llewellyn Publication, Woodbury, Minnesota 1946
83. Weiss Brian L. M.D., "Meditation. Achieving Inner Peace and Tranquility in Your Life", Hay house, Inc. Carlsbad, California 2007
84. Witkowski Waldemar, "Jam Jest", Nowator, Siedlce 2008
85. Yapko Michael D. "Podstawy hipnozy", Gdanskie Wydawnictwo Psychologiczne, Gdansk 2000

CPSIA information can be obtained
at www.ICGtesting.com
Printed in the USA
LVOW05s1946161017
552623LV00014B/739/P

9 781504 386692